The Impatient Dr. Lange

The Impatient

SEEMA YASMIN

Dr. Lange

One Man's Fight to End
the Global HIV Epidemic

Foreword by
Princess Mabel van Oranje

Fountaindale Public Library
Bolingbrook, IL
(630) 759-2102

JOHNS HOPKINS UNIVERSITY PRESS
Baltimore

Johns Hopkins University Press
2715 North Charles Street
Baltimore, Maryland 21218-4363
www.press.jhu.edu

Library of Congress Cataloging-in-Publication Data

Names: Yasmin, Seema, 1982– author.
Title: The impatient Dr. Lange : one man's fight to end the global
    HIV epidemic / Seema Yasmin ; foreword by Princess Mabel
    van Oranje
Description: Baltimore : Johns Hopkins University Press, 2018. |
    Includes index.
Identifiers: LCCN 2018002312 | ISBN 9781421426624 (pbk. : alk.
    paper) | ISBN 9781421426631 (electronic) | ISBN 1421426625 (pbk.
    : alk. paper) | ISBN 1421426633 (electronic)
Subjects: | MESH: Lange, Joep. | HIV Infections | Acquired Im-
    munodeficiency Syndrome | Anti-Retroviral Agents | Biomedical
    Research—history | History, 20th Century | History, 21st Century
    | Biography
Classification: LCC RC607.A26 | NLM WZ 100 | DDC
    362.196/9792—dc23
    LC record available at https://lccn.loc.gov/2018002312

A catalog record for this book is available from the British Library.

All illustrations courtesy of Rietje de Krieger.

*Special discounts are available for bulk purchases of this book. For
more information, please contact Special Sales at 410-516-6936 or
specialsales@press.jhu.edu.*

Johns Hopkins University Press uses environmentally friendly book
materials, including recycled text paper that is composed of at least
30 percent post-consumer waste, whenever possible.

· · · · · ·

To Khateejah, Zohra, and Yasmin—for showing me that women can do everything

To Body & Soul, the young people I met at Teen Spirit, and all those living with and affected by HIV/AIDS. You have taught me how to fight and how to love.

• • • • • •

Some people—and I am one of them—hate happy ends. We feel cheated. Harm is the norm. Doom should not jam.—Vladimir Nabokov, *Pnin*

••••••

People living deeply have no fear of death.
—Anaïs Nin, *The Diary of Anaïs Nin*, volume 2

CONTENTS

The tragedy of Malaysia Airlines flight MH17, which was shot down in the summer of 2014, left gaping holes in the families of two hundred and ninety-eight men, women, and children. For the international AIDS community, the blow was devastating. Six people committed to the fight against HIV/AIDS lost their lives on their way to the twentieth International AIDS Conference in Melbourne, Australia. Among them were my friends Dr. Joep Lange and his partner, Jacqueline van Tongeren, who had dedicated their lives to the fight against AIDS.

Joep was a pioneer in advocating for access to HIV treatment. After the introduction of antiretroviral therapy, he spearheaded a movement to make the drugs available to everyone infected with the virus—rich and poor—regardless of where they were from. He also led the first clinical trials that showed how these drugs could prevent the spread of HIV from pregnant women to their unborn children.

Joep's leadership style was fierce and honest. Joep dared to be upfront with those in power and hold them accountable for their actions, or inactions, against HIV. His words could make people uncomfortable, but they certainly spurred action. Those scientists and policy makers who believed that it was too expensive and too difficult to get antiretrovirals to sub-Saharan Africa were encouraged by one of Joep's now famous mantras: "If we can get cold Coca-Cola and beer to every remote corner of Africa, it should not be impossible to do the same with drugs." His pragmatic approach and sometimes unexpected partnerships—such as with Heineken or the army in Tanzania—were always focused on delivering results for those most in need.

HIV was more than an infectious disease to Joep. Over the years, he became acutely aware of how disease and poverty are fully interlinked. Traveling from his home in Amsterdam, Joep crisscrossed the globe visiting health facilities around the world—from HIV clinics in Kampala to hospitals in Bangkok to community test centers in rural Nigeria. Wherever he went, Joep always took the time to learn about the realities on the ground, speak with those affected, and explore innovative solutions to increase the effectiveness of interventions. He was outraged by the suffering of those who could not afford the medications that were so easily available to his patients in the Netherlands.

Joep taught us that epidemics are fueled by injustice. He was unafraid to broaden his reach beyond HIV and fight for improved access to health care in sub-Saharan Africa. When he established the PharmAccess Foundation, his goal was to provide health insurance and medicines to the poorest of the poor. Some told him his goals were too lofty. Joep ignored them and continued to push, together with Jacqueline, for improved health care for all.

Joep and Jacqueline's commitment to getting medicines into the hands of those who needed them has likely saved hundreds of thousands of lives. Even in death, their efforts continue. The PharmAccess Foundation, the Amsterdam Institute for Global Health and Development, and the Joep Lange Institute are just some of their legacies that carry on their visionary work.

Much remains to be done. Without Joep and Jacqueline's compassionate concern and leadership, we all have an obligation to step up our efforts in the fight against HIV/AIDS. Too many people are still becoming infected; too many are still losing their lives to a preventable and treatable disease.

There are many stories to be told about Joep's life as a scientist, doctor, and activist. I hope that the selection highlighted in this biography will spark a new wave of activism and inspire a new generation of scientists, doctors, policy makers, and advocates to end the AIDS epidemic. As Joep taught us, change will happen only if we make it happen.

Princess Mabel van Oranje

HOW THIS BOOK CAME TO BE

I first met Joep Lange when I was seventeen and idealistic. He seemed tall and important. Stepping away from a podium at a London conference, he collected his notebook and swept a hand over his short, graying hair. He had finished giving a talk about HIV. My mum, who was a consultant to the International AIDS Society where Joep worked, gently pushed me toward him. "Go on, go on, he will talk to you," she said. I wasn't sure.

I was cutting school regularly. Dumping my textbooks in the hallway of our east London flat, I would take the bus that went west from Hackney toward Great Ormond Street Hospital to volunteer at Body & Soul, an organization that supported families and young people living with HIV and AIDS. I started working at Body & Soul when I was fourteen. Besides counseling young people through exams, first loves, and the nasty side effects of HIV medicines, I pushed the British government for better sexual health education in schools. While I was winning national awards for my advocacy on sexual health and HIV, my teachers were calling my mum to complain about my absences.

So I didn't think Joep would talk to me. I was used to British professors with their hoity airs and graces. They looked at me through narrow eyes when I asked if I could spend time in their HIV labs. "No," they said. It would take too long to train me. It was too much of a bother.

Not Joep. He escaped a semicircle of scientists who had gathered around him near the podium, slipping through the crowd in the manner of a person adept at evading perfunctory chitchat. My mum once told me that he found small talk ghastly and would press his cell phone to his ear and pretend to be on a call to avoid it at the end of meetings. But that day he walked up to me. "I want to be like you," I blurted out. "I want to do a PhD and find a cure for AIDS." Joep smiled. He bent his neck, bringing his face closer to mine, and said, "If you want to help people, first you need to learn how to take care of them. Go to medical school."

So I did.

I knew Joep was a scientist, but I hadn't realized he was a doctor. I thought doctors worked in clinics and saw patients every day. I thought they cared for individuals, not for populations. I didn't know that a doctor could save thousands of lives in one swoop by making a jab at a government official or by berating drug companies, pushing them to slash the cost of their medicines. I didn't understand those things or discover public health until I met Joep.

Standing next to Joep as he told me to go to medical school was Dr. Charles Boucher, a Dutch virologist and a world expert on HIV resistance. Charles looked like a mad scientist from a comic book. He wore round spectacles, and a halo of brown curls sprouted from his head and seemed to stand on end. As Joep helped to plan my career, Charles invited me to spend a summer in his virology lab in Utrecht. For three glorious months, I ate pickled herring and laced petri dishes with a mouse version of the virus that causes SARS. It was in a Dutch lab that I learned to pipette and make gels, to watch as viruses outwit the drugs designed to kill them. I saw how discoveries made on a lab bench end up at a patient's bedside.

I went to medical school on Joep's advice, and I wrote this book because of Charles. Joep's legacy needs to be shared, Charles said on a phone call from Amsterdam in 2016, as I packed up my house in Dallas to move to Washington, DC. I was on my third career. I had switched from working as a hospital doctor in England to being a disease detective in the US government's Epidemic Intelligence Service, then trained as a journalist at the University of Toronto.

I was working as a newspaper reporter for the *Dallas Morning News* and as a professor of epidemiology at the University of Texas at Dallas when Charles called. I was looking for a change. A tornado had ripped through my home the previous year while my family was inside and while I was in Liberia reporting on the Ebola epidemic.

I planned to freelance from Washington and to begin a memoir about my life as a disease detective. I was scared to write about Joep, fearful of reducing a complicated man to a one-dimensional scientist. News stories about him read like hagiographies. I knew they were imprecise.

I told Charles I would work on a book proposal—but I didn't. I left it for months, and then, standing on the porch of a log cabin at the Playa writer's residency in rural Oregon, watching oily muskrats glide through the water while birds skimmed the surface of an expansive white salt plain behind them, I appreciated that I might not be there, might not be writing a memoir about my life as a doctor, were it not for Joep. He saw ambition and drive in a seventeen-year-old, and instead of saying it would be hard to follow in his footsteps or that I should focus on my immediate studies, he made the impossible seem possible.

Joep presumed that a girl raised by a single parent from an immigrant Muslim community—a community where girls were raised to be house-wives, where few people went to university, and none had been to medical school—could be a doctor. And I believed him. That short conversation transformed my life.

The day Joep died I was two weeks into my job at the *Dallas Morning News* and about to go live on CNN to discuss a front-page story I had written the previous day. It was about children as young as six years old crossing the border from Mexico into Texas alone and the outraged politicians who were claiming the children were filthy and bringing diseases—even Ebola—into America. I wrote that the children were more likely to pick up infections in Texas than they were in Central America.

"You're off the hook," a CNN producer told me moments before we were meant to go live. "We've got breaking news. A jetliner has crashed in the Ukraine."

Then my mum phoned. "Joep is on that plane. He was going to the AIDS conference in Australia. I'm so sorry, Seema." I walked quickly toward the bathroom but didn't make it before my face was wet with tears. The newspaper's managing editor walked past and asked why pieces of tissue were stuck to my cheeks. I pointed to the television screens lining the walls of the newsroom. He put his hands over his mouth.

Sitting next to Joep on Malaysia Airlines flight MH17 was Jacqueline van Tongeren, Joep's partner in life, love, and the fight against AIDS. Jacqueline was an AIDS nurse who baffled me when I was a teenager be-cause she had owned art galleries, danced ballet, and restored historical buildings—all before she was thirty. I wasn't sure how one woman could encompass so many talents.

Some of her friends told me they were glad, in a way, that Jacqueline was on the plane. She would not have been able to cope without her love. They imagined the pair died how they lived—holding each other close.

As a journalist, I feel bound to declare my relationship with Joep at the beginning of this book. Our meetings were brief and infrequent—over the years I saw Joep and Jacqueline a handful of times at AIDS conferences around the world. Despite this and despite his schedule—hopping on and off planes, traveling continents, and often missing flights—Joep wrote letters of recommendation for me, even when I was applying for opportunities way out of my league. He never questioned a driven person's ability to achieve everything. He once began a lecture, addressing a room full of stodgy professors, with a quote by the Queen of Hearts from Lewis Carroll's *Alice in Wonderland:* "Why, sometimes I've believed as many as six impossible things before breakfast."

Journalists talk a lot about balance. I'm not sure there is such a thing. I knew Joep, and that colors my view of him, but I have strived to present a complicated man in all his complexity. Joep was kind and compassionate, he cared deeply about his patients and about confronting injustice. Joep could be difficult to work with. He raged against HIV, and that fury spilled into his relationships. He made my mum cry after a meeting of AIDS experts in Seattle because he was impatient at the progress of a project they were working on together. Nothing was ever quite fast enough.

A few people I interviewed told me that long friendships with him disintegrated after quarrels over seemingly minor things. Others shared stories of astonishing tenderness and spoke of a man who eschewed ego to protect others.

Jacqueline was quite different. Through more than fifty interviews and countless hours spent sifting through records, I found not one negative word uttered or written about her. She seemed to be universally adored.

Interviews for this book took place in person in Amsterdam, Den Haag, Barcelona, Boston, Washington, DC, London, Pretoria, and Cape Town, and via telephone and Skype with Joep's and Jacqueline's family, friends, and colleagues in Australia, Uganda, France, the United States, Thailand, South Africa, and Argentina. I visited Joep's childhood home in a village that no longer exists. I talked to Joep's and Jacqueline's friends and families, their colleagues from the 1980s and 1990s as well as the people they spoke to in the days before they died. I constructed scenes from these interviews and from written records, medical journals, and recorded discussions. I interviewed experts in Dutch history and those who study the Dutch AIDS response to learn how the country's past—its religious wars and imperialist legacy—shaped a man who became a global leader in the fight against AIDS.

I am grateful for those who talked through tears and shared private memories. Most of all, I am grateful to Joep's sister, Riet, and his only son, Max, for their generosity in sharing their brother and father.

This book was written in the spring and summer of 2017, around the third anniversary of flight MH17's crash. Two hundred and ninety-eight people died that July day, among them babies and teachers, grandparents and scientists. This book is for all of them.

The Impatient Dr. Lange

1 *The End*

The plane would crash in six hours, and his face would be on the news. American television anchors would mangle his Dutch name, stretching and shortening the "o" and the "e" into swooping ooo's and snappy a's as they described him: genius scientist, AIDS fighter, medical diplomat, father of five, humanitarian, mastermind of a potential cure for HIV. Dr. Joseph Marie Albert Lange, better known as Joep—pronounced Yoop— was dead, and the world wondered if the cure for HIV lay singed and scattered across a field in the Ukraine.

The rebels had shot down the wrong plane. Joep, who was known for publicly cursing out fools even when those fools were presidents and Nobel Prize winners, probably muttered "stupid" and "God verdomme" in Dutch from seat 3C in flight MH17's business class as the plane was pierced by shrapnel. A Buk ground-to-air missile fired by pro-Russian separatists had exploded near its nose.

Damn those idiots fighting a bloody war with Russia. Damn the air traffic controllers for flying his plane into a war zone.

Joep didn't even like Malaysia Airlines. He had racked up millions of miles on his favorite airline, KLM, as he flew around the world chasing a viral epidemic. But Malaysia Airlines flight MH17 offered the cheapest business class tickets from Amsterdam to Melbourne, where he was headed to speak at the twentieth International AIDS Conference.

Sixteen thousand people waited for him in Melbourne, waited to hear the Dutch doctor with the soft voice and the words that cut like knives. Joep spoke his mind. He didn't hide behind jargon or politics. He had put his neck on the line since the very beginning of the epidemic—which coincided with the beginning of his career—by advocating for the poor and the vulnerable, taking positions his peers called fanciful and absurd. On the highest platforms, at the biggest AIDS conferences, Joep disagreed with the world's top scientists and refused to settle for the status quo—a status quo that favored the white and the wealthy.

He called scientists and policy makers cowards and imbeciles when they said it was too difficult to get lifesaving AIDS drugs to Africans. "If we can get cold Coca-Cola and beer to every remote corner of Africa, surely we can do the same with drugs," was his mantra.

Joep first met AIDS in the summer of 1981. He was twenty-six years old, fresh out of medical school, and about to come face to face with a new and mysterious killer. The men who walked into the emergency room of his Amsterdam hospital, their bodies feverish, their eyes glassy and rimmed with blue-gray circles, were the same age as he, sometimes younger. Walking corpses collapsed onto gurneys, their bodies rattled with an infection so new to humanity that there was no primer for battling it.

The virus floating through their veins, burrowing into their brains, and making its home in their glands had jumped from monkeys to humans, morphing and mutating along the way. It attacked the immune system, the very part of the body designed to keep intruders at bay. Joep's patients were left wide open to a slew of bizarre infections that grew inside their lungs and crept beneath their skin. The young men with hollowed-out eyes coughed raspy coughs and sat in pools of diarrhea. They died slow, drawn-out deaths.

There was no dignity in AIDS, only bewilderment. Young lovers were left bereft, parents were dazed. Joep rolled up his sleeves and got to work pressing his palms into bellies, asking his young patients questions about sex and desire. He packed his bags with novels and notepads and flew to San Francisco, London, and Sydney to talk to doctors who said their patients were dying of the same plague and there was nothing they could do to save them.

AIDS was a guaranteed death sentence back then—Joep helped to change that. He ran from the ward to the lab clutching vials of his patients' blood in his long fingers, the tails of his white coat flapping as he hurried along the corridors of the University of Amsterdam's Academic Medical Center. This new disease couldn't be battled at the bedside alone. He needed to be at the lab bench, interrogating the virus that caused AIDS.

Switching between stethoscope and microscope, petri dishes and patients, Joep stripped HIV to its bare bones, revealing the virus's anatomy and deciphering its Achilles' heel. While working on his PhD in the mid-1980s, he made seminal discoveries about HIV and AIDS. Over the next thirty years, he published close to four hundred articles and saved, by some estimates, millions of lives.

When Joep stepped onto the Malaysia Airlines plane on July 17, 2014, he was beside the love of his life, Jacqueline van Tongeren, a woman who had embraced half a dozen careers before she embraced him. Jacqueline was the picture of elegance, shiny brown hair swept her shoulders, couture frocks swished around her calves. High cheekbones and smooth skin belied her sixty-four—soon to be sixty-five—years. Jacqueline's birthday was just nine days away. Joep would turn sixty in September.

They had met on the AIDS ward of the University of Amsterdam's Academic Medical Center in 1990, when she was hired as head nurse. Jacqueline was in a relationship back then, and Joep was married to the mother of his five children. Eventually, their decades-long friendship bloomed into a love affair that they announced to knowing friends and family seven years before their deaths.

Jacqueline sat upright in 3A, the window seat next to Joep, her posture honed from years of dancing ballet. She eyed Malaysia Airlines' business class menu and texted her friend, Han Nefkens, that she was excited to taste the delicious Asian food that reminded her of Indonesia, where she was born. She had already emailed her brother to share some important news.

The night before she boarded flight MH17, Jacqueline prepared her will. Her younger brother, Philip "Flip" van Tongeren, was the executor. "I meant to call you to tell you," she wrote in an email she sent him at one a.m.

There was another secret to share. After years of living apart, the pair had purchased a new home together—a love nest. They would move in when they got back from Melbourne in ten days. Joep planned to write a novel there, Jacqueline hoped to use it as a base while they traveled around the world spending month-long stints in their dream destinations. Of course, they would never stop battling the HIV epidemic. They had seen up close how a virus could creep into bodies and destroy white blood cells, then jump across borders and crush economies.

Now the air above a Ukrainian village was choked with smoke and regret. Guidebooks to the Australian outback turned to cinder, the faces of koala bears crumpled and burned. Travel toothbrushes melted into plastic puddles among stalks of scorched, yellow grass. The wrecked body of the plane lay strewn across the field, jagged pieces of its belly and tail still smoldering.

Every person on board was dead. Two hundred and ninety-eight Australians, Indonesians, Malaysians, Brits, Dutch, Germans, Belgians, Filipinos, with one American, one Canadian, and one New Zealander. Among the dead: three babies, seventy-seven children, a nun, a helicopter pilot, five AIDS researchers. An Australian couple who lost their son and daughter-in-law on another Malaysia Airlines plane, flight MH370, when it disappeared in March that year, lost their granddaughter on flight MH17. Bodies rained down over houses and fields. Their limbs and lives became bargaining chips for pro-Russian separatists.

But death was still six hours away. It was a cool summer morning in Amsterdam and Jacqueline was crouching on the floor of her apartment, cramming Missoni skirts and Comme des Garcons blouses into a suitcase already stuffed with shoes. She texted her best friend, Peggy van Leeuwen: "I'm like the Imelda Marcos of Holland!"

Joep was shooting off a sarcastic email to one of his staffers, squeezing medical journals and three novels into a laptop bag to read on the plane, then looping a leash around his diabetic Irish terrier's neck. He stroked Lizzy's soft gray fur. They stepped onto Beethovenstraat, the tony street he lived on with his children, for a stroll before the long flight. The air was fresh, Lizzy was weaving in and out of his legs. He waved at a friend driving past them.

2 *Origin Stories*

It was a breezy morning in August 1961 when a teenaged boy stepped onto a merchant ship in the Oslofjord docks in Norway. Arne Vidar Røed had just turned fifteen and earned a job as a kitchen hand aboard the *Hoegh Aronde*, a four-thousand-ton cargo ship.

It was Arne's first day as a sailor. What could be more thrilling to a teenaged boy than leaving behind the frosty waters of Scandinavia and floating toward the warm waves of the Gulf of Guinea?

Ship life bore its own tedium. Restless from months marooned on the metal vessel with only men for companionship, Arne was ready for adventure. He stepped off the ship in Douala, Cameroon's largest city, and found it heaving with the traffic of hard-working people—fishermen, ship makers, farmers—people who used the strength of their bodies to make a living.

Ramshackle bars wafted sweat and the sounds of *bikutsi* music through the streets. Arne knocked back beer and stomped his feet with a new friend who taught him how to thrust his hips in time to the beat. When he boarded the ship days later, he carried with him a souvenir from that night. It was gonorrhea, the first of three sexually transmitted infections he acquired on his virgin voyage.

Arne sailed north with his new microbial companion, stepping ashore at ports in Nigeria, Ghana, Côte d'Ivoire, Liberia, Guinea, and Senegal. It would be ten months before he returned home to Norway, another four years before a nameless parasite inside his veins would flow to the surface.

In the meantime, with his infectious memento still buried deep inside him, the merchant seaman sailed to Canada, the Caribbean, Asia, and Europe. Besides a two-day stop in Mombasa, Kenya, in the mid-1960s, Arne never returned to Africa.

In 1965, Arne settled down in Oslo, married, and had a baby girl. By the time his second daughter was born in 1966, the young father's joints were swollen and hot, his chest was tight and congested, and his muscles ached deeply. The glands beneath Arne's jaw were tender, throbbing knots. Angry lumps poked out along the creases of his groin and in his armpits. Crops of red blisters dotted his chest and back.

Arne's doctors were baffled. In an Oslo clinic, they listed the young man's maladies and scratched their heads. Occam's razor is a philosophical law applied to medicine. It guides a doctor to link every one of the patient's problems to a single unifying diagnosis. But what would explain a cough, fever, strange rashes, swollen lymph nodes, and aching joints? Perhaps Hickam's dictum, the counterargument to Occam's law of parsimony, was at play. Hickam's dictum states that patients can have as many different diseases as they please. Yes, that was it.

The doctors gave Arne a vague and useless diagnosis of a connective tissue disorder. They scribbled a prescription instructing the pharmacist to dispense steroid pills. They hoped this would dampen the immune system's rage.

Then Arne's wife fell sick. Minor urinary tract infections flared into major diseases of her bladder and kidneys. Her tongue sprouted a furry coat of white fungus, her brain swelled against her skull. She was diagnosed with leukemia.

Arne's symptoms waxed and waned. Too sick to sail, he took on work as a truck driver delivering cargo across the Netherlands, Austria, Germany, and France. His two eldest children were happy, healthy girls, but when his youngest daughter turned two she fell sick with bizarre infections rarely seen in children. Her lungs bloomed with the same white fungus that coated her mother's tongue. The spores refused to budge, even though her parents fed her spoonfuls of a gloopy, pink, antifungal syrup.

Bacteria invaded the little girl's body—her joints, bones, and blood were colonized with *Staphylococcus aureus* and *Haemophilus influenzae*. Then a virus attacked. Varicella-zoster, the bug that causes chickenpox and shingles, spread through her organs killing her before her third birthday.

The grieving father groaned beneath the pains in his hips and knees. Swellings and rashes continued to flare up and down his body. At twenty-nine years old, Arne became incontinent, soiling his trousers throughout the day. When he went to visit the doctors again, they watched as he hobbled through the clinic hallways. His legs were becoming paralyzed. Arne babbled like a madman. The doctors scribbled "dementia" and "unknown etiology" in his medical notes.

Arne died three months after his youngest daughter's death. It was April 1976, three months before his thirtieth birthday. His wife died in December, leaving doctors triply perplexed. Dr. Stig Fredrik Frøland, a physician at the National Hospital in Norway, cut open their bodies and pulled out organs riddled with fungi, bacteria, and viruses. Their spinal cords dripped pus, their spleens were withered, their immune systems massacred.

No doctor could name the illness or explain why the trio had suffered fulminant deaths. One Norwegian doctor had an idea. He took it to Italy. At a meeting of the Italian-Scandinavian neuropathological society in Rome in 1977, Dr. Christian Fredrik Lindboe, a colleague of Dr. Frøland, presented the unusual cases.

He clicked through slides of the young girl's lymphoid tissue, her father's brain, her mother's spleen. He showed their nerve cells mangled by an unknown attacker, their T helper cells all but vanished. To the room of neurologists and pathologists, he dared to pose a hypothesis: perhaps an infectious agent—a virus—was responsible for their deaths. Dr. Lindboe was right, but it would be eleven years before he could prove it.

In 1987, he went back to the hospital's freezers with Dr. Frøland, thawed the family's archived blood samples, and searched their remains for a peculiar virus making the news. Thousands had died from a plague that was spreading across the globe, and now there was a way to test for the new infection. They tested the samples. Arne, his wife, and their daughter were positive for the human immunodeficiency virus.

"But in science as in other aspects of life, timing is important," Dr. Lindboe said. "And we were definitely too early this time."

Arne's aching hands may have steered his cargo truck up and down the flat roads of northern Holland into the hills of southern Holland in 1971, just as a lanky, softly spoken seventeen-year-old boy was hatching his own plans to escape provincial life and embark on an international voyage.

Joseph Marie Albert Lange, known to everyone as Joep, lived in the town of Den Briel, its name derived from the Celtic word *brogilo*, meaning "closed off." The teenager wanted desperately to get out.

His life had been a series of moves to increasingly larger towns. Joep was born in 1954 in Nieuwenhagen, a bucolic coal-mining village in the southern tip of the country, where life revolved around the pair of imposing Catholic churches a few hundred yards from his house.

Nieuwenhagen sat in Limburg, the Netherlands' southernmost province and the only part of the country that wasn't flat. Joep's birthplace was home to some of the best chocolate and beer in Holland, but it was deeply Catholic and claustrophobic.

On a map of the Netherlands, Limburg juts out of the mainland like a polyp on a stalk, burying itself into Germany on the east and Belgium on the west. Brussels and Cologne were closer to Joep's hometown than the country's own capital, Amsterdam. Up north, the city folk looked down on their southern neighbors and their singsongy dialect of Limburgish, with its mishmash of German, Dutch, and Flemish.

During the Eighty Years' War, which began in the mid-sixteenth century, the Netherlands fought for its independence from Spain. Limburg was home to many bloody battles, but Limburgians, most of whom were staunch Catholics, often chose to fight against the Calvinist Hollanders in the north siding instead with the Spaniards, who were Catholic. The

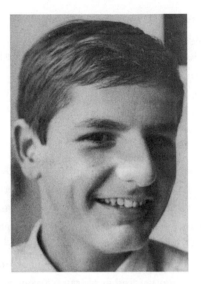

Joseph Marie Albert Lange,
known to everyone as Joep

province continued sending its young men to fight on the side of the Germans up until the 1860s.

Always the outsiders, many Limburgers considered themselves distinct from their brethren in the north, reluctantly celebrating Queen's Day and backing their nation in the World Cup. Every other day, they were Limburgians first and Dutch second.

Despite Limburg's strong Catholic tradition, Joep's family eschewed the influence of the Church as much as they could. When she was told by a priest to have more children, Joep's maternal grandmother, Maria, told the man to hush and stop interfering in her business.

Maria married Sjeng Bertram, who also came from a large Catholic family. The couple were self-made entrepreneurs, opening a café in Nieuwenhagen during World War II where American soldiers chugged beer and chatted with Dutch women. Twice a week they converted the annex into a dance hall.

Business was good, and with the help of their daughter—whom they named after the holy mother—and her husband, Sjef Reumkens, they bought one of the largest villas in the village, hoping to hear the pitter patter of tiny feet across the tiled floors. Villa Belvedere was a stunning brick building shaded by oak and spar trees, set back from the road behind a wooden fence.

The younger Maria and her husband, Sjef, had two children in the early years of the war, a son named Jean, and a daughter named Maria, who was known as Marietje and Rietje, or Riet, to avoid confusion in a household filled with three Marias.

When Riet was eight months old her father, Sjef, fell ill and was diagnosed with a brain aneurysm. He remained sickly throughout Riet and Jean's childhood, suffering paralysis until his death at the age of forty. The children were not yet ten years old.

Maria's friends stepped in to help the young widow find a new beau. A few years after the loss of her husband, they invited Maria to a party in Nieuwenhagen and introduced her to a dashing man ten years her junior. Joseph Lange, known as Joep, came from a middle-class family in nearby Heerlen and worked as an engineer at the Oranje Nassau coal mine.

It was love at first sight. Their age difference—a scandal in a small, conservative village—was spoken about in hushed tones. The pair courted, married, and had a son within a year. Keeping with the family tradition of passing down names, they christened their son, Joseph Marie Albert Lange. The child was born in the villa on September 25, 1954. Joep's older siblings, Riet and Jean, cooed over their baby brother while the grandparents fussed around him.

When American soldiers liberated Limburg, Joep's grandparents converted the annex that was a dance hall into a small movie theater and eventually built a big movie theater in the center of Nieuwenhagen by Joep's third birthday. But the timing was unfortunate. Television sets were popping up in homes across Holland. The grandparents moved into an apartment above the ill-fated movie theater, and Joep's mother, seeking independence from her parents and their cooped-up quarters,

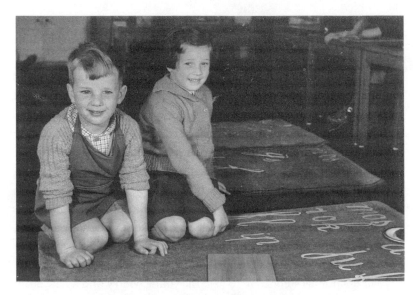

Joep with his older sister, Rietje de Krieger

suggested to her husband that they move to Heerlen, the town three miles away where he worked. She was thrilled when he said yes. Heerlen meant relief from living under the same roof as her parents.

Joep's father was an opinionated man who stoked intellectual debates at the dinner table. Joep learned to speak his mind and hold his ground. Still, he couldn't talk his way out of the Catholic school that his mother insisted he attend. The Heerlen school was run by Franciscan monks who walked the long corridors in drab, brown robes and sandals and scolded the children for any manner of disobedience.

Joep's mother held on loosely to some Catholic beliefs, but his father had renounced religion as a child when his mother had died. Joep Sr. was an altar boy at the time of his mother's death. He found himself unable to reconcile his loss with his faith and became an atheist. Like his father, Joep thought religion was nonsense, especially when it got in the way of his favorite pastime—reading.

The literature selection at his Catholic school was paltry, and one day

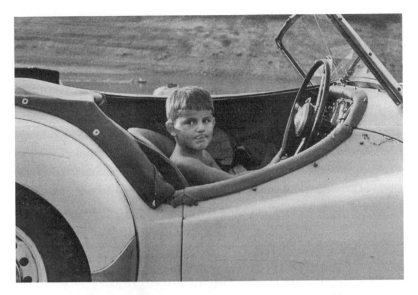

Joep, as a child, in the driver's seat of a convertible

Joep announced his literary dismay to the monks, telling them that the local library offered a far superior selection of books. They slapped him.

Books were his entry point into a world outside the provincial Netherlands. Vladimir Nabokov transported him to Russia and the Ivy League colleges of the United States; Gustave Flaubert introduced him to scandal in the French countryside. Joep buried himself in volumes of Dutch, English, and French prose. Eastern European writers were his favorite: he read and reread Dutch translations of Nikolai Gogol. He devoured books by Willem Elsschot.

Some days Riet struggled to get into Joep's bedroom because piles of books were stacked against his bedroom walls, scattered around his bed and blocking the doorway. He dreamed of becoming a novelist, and over dinner one day he announced his career plans to his family.

"I'm going to be a writer," Joep said.

"But how will you earn a living?" said Maria.

The boy thought for a moment, then his sister came to his rescue.

"Maybe you could be a writer and a doctor," said Riet. She reminded him of his beloved author, J. Slauerhoff, the Dutch poet and novelist who graduated from the University of Amsterdam's medical school. He wrote fiction and worked as a ship's doctor.

The boy's eyes widened.

If he did go to medical school, Joep would become the first doctor in the family. He had an aunt on his father's side who worked as a medical missionary in Africa, where she nursed sick coal miners. On trips back to the Netherlands she sat Joep in her lap and told him stories about the squalid living conditions of her patients, who worked in the mines, mines like the one his father managed.

When Joep turned eleven, the Dutch government announced the end of coal mining, and his father was forced to look for work elsewhere. He found work at Oxirane, a chemical plant in Den Briel, a seaport one hundred and fifty miles northwest of Heerlen. The town was bombed in World War II and undergoing a construction boom when the family moved.

At school, Joep's accent was mocked by his classmates. "Wat blieft?" he enquired politely when they asked him to repeat a word. But his courteous way of asking what they were saying only fueled the bullies. "Wat blieft?" they sneered, collapsing into fits of laughter. They were tickled by the country boy's melodic sentences and southern accent. Joep couldn't roll his r's like a northerner, and he spoke with soft, oily g's that emanated from his mouth, not the harsh, guttural g's that vibrated in the throats of the kids from Den Briel.

He wanted to leave. Vladimir Nabokov enjoyed long stints in London and Berlin before planting roots in America; Elsschot left Antwerp for Paris. If Joep was to write great literature he needed to get out of the Netherlands. Academic excellence was his escape route.

In the summer of 1971, Joep found liberation in good grades and an international exchange program that took him to Robinson High School in Tampa, Florida, for a year. The boy from the Dutch village became an American high school student: exciting for him, painful for the close-knit family he left behind. His parents and siblings wrote him long letters, since international phone calls were expensive.

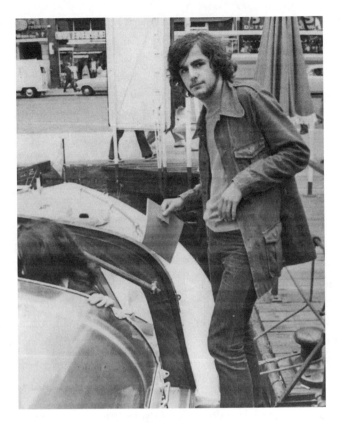

Young Joep

But at Christmastime, Joep called Riet on the phone. His host father had lost his job and couldn't afford to feed another mouth. "You have to call the organization and tell them to find you a new family," Riet said. A journalism professor, Dean McClendon, took him into his home in Temple Terrace, where Joep shared a bunk bed with Dean's son and gifted his daughter, Tricia, the Beatles' White Album for her thirteenth birthday.

Joep had already completed high school in Den Briel. Tampa was for fun. He found school easy and excelled in literature and the sciences. He was curious and appreciated the methodical steps of science experiments with their controls and diligent note-taking. Medicine intrigued him with its mix of science and human stories. Perhaps he would be the next Anton Chekhov, Mikhail Bulgakov, or Sir Arthur Conan Doyle—that rare figure who dazzled both the literary and medical worlds.

Literature offered the constant escape he needed when he felt stifled and bored—which was often. Joep joined Robinson High School's Quill and Scroll literary club and danced with homecoming queen Donna Seville at prom.

"Here you see an intellectual at work," Joep wrote in the yearbook beneath a photo of himself, his hair grazing his shoulders. It was a note to his classmate David Booker. "He is handsome. And he hopes to see you at his home. And that is Holland. My dear Holland."

He wore his black hair in a shaggy bob like Bob Dylan, one of his two favorite American musicians. The other was Frank Zappa. He liked the way the musician combined activism with art and poked fun at American culture. Joep owned more than forty of Zappa's records.

When he returned to Den Briel in 1972, Riet thought he looked like a Dutch Provo, a member of the counterculture movement born in Holland in the 1960s. Provos believed in a nonviolent uprising against the establishment, and her brother was, after all, antihierarchical, antireligion, straight to the point, and determined.

When he applied to medical school in Amsterdam in the 1970s, Dutch universities were transitioning from elitist institutions to democratically run organizations where students and professors were considered equals. Joep applied to the University of Amsterdam, a left-wing bulwark with ties to the Communist Party.

The city was going through a revolution. Amsterdam was developing a reputation for being hip, drug-friendly, and a must-see stop on the international hippy trail. At the same time the city was collapsing—literally. Built on swamps, Amsterdam's foundations were rotting and homes built quickly and cheaply in the 1920s and 1930s were disintegrating. The woongroep movement, which believed in communal living and the occupation of derelict homes, was taking off.

This is the Amsterdam that Joep moved to in 1972 at the age of eighteen. He entered medical school imagining that the profession would support his career as a writer. For the first year, he lived in east Amsterdam, sharing a room in a house owned by two elderly ladies, but he wasn't keen on the accommodations.

During his second year of medical school, immersed in skeletons and Nabokov novels, Joep was roused from his books by devastating news. His father had suffered a stroke. Joep Sr. was only forty-six. Joep rushed to Den Briel to be with his parents. His mother was distraught and fearful of losing another young husband.

Joep Sr. survived the bleeding in his brain, but he was not the same man. Less opinionated, confused, he was even paralyzed for a short while. The stroke stripped him of his memory and wit, and he was forced to give up the work he enjoyed. Maria moved them back to Limburg.

Joep returned to Amsterdam and buried himself in his studies. Anxious about his father's health and worried about his mother's strength, he was unaware that in Norway another family was suffering its own medical misfortune. As Joep was rotating through clinics in rheumatology and cardiology, Arne's bones were growing weaker and his fevers flaring to new heights.

While Joep was being counseled by his professors not to take up a career in the "dying field" of infectious disease, Arne was burying his daughter. The two-year-old's body was riddled with unexplained infections.

Joep's professors insisted that antibiotics had cured all the major infections and that there were no new discoveries to be made in the field of microbiology. They advised him to specialize in cardiology.

Then, two years before Joep graduated as a doctor, his father died suddenly of a heart attack at the age of fifty-two. Joep was distraught and discombobulated. The kind, charming man from whom he had inherited his sense of humor, eloquence, and atheism had left him.

He went to live with his sister in Baarn, a short train ride away from Amsterdam. It was in Riet's cozy kitchen that he met Thomas Rap, a publisher whose children attended the same school as Riet's daughters.

Enthralled by the publisher's proximity to literature, Joep moved into the shed at the bottom of Thomas's garden in Bunschoten. The town was more than an hour away from Amsterdam, and the rickety wooden shed let in the cold air, but it was worth the long commute and the freezing nights to come home to a house where literature flowed into every nook and cranny, a real *salon littéraire*. Writers converged around tables and argued about prose over red wine. Riet knew her little brother was suffering the cold for his love of literature. One night she drove to Thomas's house, her back seats piled with thick blankets that would keep her little brother warm in his literary grotto.

Thomas and Joep were often engrossed in animated debates about Slauerhoff and Elsschot, Nabokov and Gogol. They stopped only to take silent breaks in the garden, where they passed each other binoculars and watched birds. Thomas was an amateur ornithologist, and Joep liked to pretend he was his student.

When he graduated from medical school in the spring of 1981, Joep wasn't aware that a strange plague was spreading across the globe, that before the droves of gay men began dying in San Francisco and Los Angeles, there had been a Norwegian family tormented by a virus so new it was nameless. Arne was one of the earliest confirmed cases of HIV in the world. His daughter is one of the first known cases of pediatric AIDS.

Human histories are strangely intertwined. The Norwegian sailor and the Dutch medical student would never meet, but Joep would spend his life immersed in the virus coursing through that sailor's blood, retracing his watery steps in search of a cure for AIDS.

"The origin of the AIDS virus is of no importance to science today," said Dr. David Heymann in 1992. At the time, Heymann was chief of research at the Global Programme on AIDS at the World Health Organization in Geneva. He was speaking to *Rolling Stone* reporter Tom Curtis, who quoted David in a March 1992 story titled "The Origin of AIDS: A Startling New Theory Attempts to Answer the Question 'Was It an Act of God or an Act of Man?'"

That startling new theory alleged that HIV was spread through a polio vaccination campaign in central Africa. A batch of vaccines was contaminated with the virus, proponents of the theory said. According to this doctrine, medicine itself seeded the global pandemic.

The mass vaccination program in question was run by Dr. Hilary Koprowski, a Polish-American researcher who, separately from Jonas Salk and Albert Sabin, had invented his own polio vaccine. It was tested in the Belgian Congo, Burundi, and Rwanda in the late 1950s and by some estimates up to seventy thousand children parted their lips and tilted back their heads for the drip drop of his oral vaccine.

Supporters of the tainted vaccine theory argued that Dr. Koprowski's polio vaccine was made using kidney cells from chimps infected with an ape version of HIV. Hearing these allegations, the Congo-based Wistar Institute, where the vaccine was manufactured, held an independent investigation. In their report, scientists said, "It can be stated with almost complete certainty that the large polio vaccine trial begun in 1957 in the Congo was not the origin of AIDS."

Dr. Koprowski's lawyers filed a lawsuit against *Rolling Stone* magazine, claiming defamation. A year after Tom Curtis's story ran, his editors printed an update. In the December 9, 1993, edition of the magazine, they wrote: "Rolling Stone regrets any damage to Dr. Koprowski's reputation that may have been caused by the article and believes this clarification sets the record straight." They were not accusing him of singlehandedly starting the AIDS epidemic.

Still, some ran with the idea. Most notably, English journalist Edward Hooper, who wrote a tome on the origins of HIV, *The River*, published in 1999. Hooper's claims were largely disputed, but he believed that samples of Dr. Koprowski's vaccine tested by the independent committee at the Wistar Institute were not the same samples that were used in the African vaccination campaign. The committee only tested samples sent from the United States, he said.

In a 2004 entry on his website, Hooper wrote: "It becomes correspondingly harder for alternative views and information to emerge in the scientific literature. Quite simply, there are a lot of scientists (many of them quite eminent ones) who find it easier to look the other way, and pretend that the [oral polio vaccine] theory has been refuted. It should be added that quite powerful forces (legal, financial and governmental) are now being invoked to further that end."

It's no wonder that alternative theories about the spread of HIV thrive, reproduce, and spread—much like the virus. Given the bloody history of unethical medical experimentation on children, the elderly, communities of color, and the poor, why would people trust doctors and the government with their health? Why wouldn't they think something as nefarious as the deliberate infection of a community could take place?

The US government continues to provide ample material to bolster conspiracy theories. Doctors from the federal government purposefully infected Guatemalan orphans and prisoners with gonorrhea beginning in 1946 and left African American men to suffer with untreated syphilis in Tuskegee for forty years. Mexican women who went to give birth at the Los Angeles County–USC clinic in in the 1960s and 1970s were sterilized without consent as part of American eugenics programs that scholars say inspired the Nazis. Across the country, more than thirty states ran federally funded programs that rendered thousands of poor women, usually women of color, unable to have children. The North Carolina Eugenics Board forcibly sterilized up to seven thousand mostly African American women and girls, some as young as nine years of age. Beginning in 2011, the US government watched for more than three years as poor, Black children sipped on lead-poisoned tap water in Flint, Michigan.

Even when intentions have been benevolent, public health campaigns have gone horribly wrong. In April 1955, nearly a quarter of a million children in the western and midwestern United States were given Salk's polio vaccine, which had been developed the previous year. But batches of the vaccine made in Cutter Laboratories, a California-based manufacturer, contained live virus because the lab's viral deactivation process had gone awry. Forty thousand children were infected with polio, two hundred were paralyzed, ten children died.

Around the same time as the Cutter incident, different batches of polio vaccine were tainted with a virus called SV40. SV40 is endemic in rhesus macaques, monkeys whose kidney cells are used in the vaccine manufacture process. The virus has been linked to higher rates of bone tumors and mesothelioma in some animals, but not in humans.

There are many more incidents. In 1901, nine children in New Jersey died when they were given smallpox vaccine contaminated with tetanus bacillus. In 1998, a rotavirus vaccine was found to cause a thirtyfold increase in intussusception, a condition where a child's bowel telescopes into itself. A year later, the manufacturer removed the vaccine from the market.

The legacy of these medical tragedies and unethical studies endures. A 2016 outbreak of tuberculosis in Marion, Alabama, prompted frustration that those affected or at risk of contracting tuberculosis were not willing to see a doctor. The town is a two-hour drive from Tuskegee, home of the Tuskegee Study of Untreated Syphilis in the Negro Male, an experiment where Black men left untreated with syphilis passed the bacteria on to their wives and unborn babies before dying slow, demented deaths themselves.

The history of mistreatment and malicious experimentation on Black bodies makes it difficult to test new treatments on diverse groups of people. Clinical trials still recruit mostly white people, even in ethnically diverse parts of the world, which makes it tricky to extrapolate clinical trial data to the many people of color who will use the medicines being tested.

History is important in understanding the spread of diseases and the stories told about them. But like Heymann in the 1990s, some doctors prefer not to dwell on the origins of HIV. Some call it a distraction from the day-to-day challenges of managing the illness. What use is a story about a fifteenth-century chimpanzee when your sickly young patient is coughing up phlegm streaked with blood and tuberculosis?

But origin stories are helpful, not just for predicting the next pandemic, but because understanding HIV's beginnings may lead us to its ending.

Deciphering what HIV looked like at its inception and comparing that with the many mutated faces of the virus today could help us find which parts of the virus have stayed the same. These parts might be small, but they would make wonderful targets for a vaccine.

HIV could have been an ancient virus carried by our ancestors. Some viruses infected humans hundreds and thousands of years ago, potentially causing pandemics. Researchers try to piece together those bygone outbreaks by analyzing the remnants of old viruses.

Where do they find these viral leftovers? Inside humans. Your DNA isn't fully human. Almost a tenth of your genome contains the instructions—not for making skin cells or eyelashes or a healthy liver—but for making viruses.

Eight percent of "human" DNA is viral. Scientists discovered around forty fragments of DNA inserted into the human genome by viruses that may have infected our ancestors up to six hundred thousand years ago.

On the tip of your X chromosome is the entire DNA of an ancient virus. This fragment, dubbed Xq21, was first noticed by researchers at Tufts University School of Medicine in 2015.

It was a startling discovery. Never had we seen the entire genetic code of a virus inserted into the human genome. Perched on chromosome X, it's as if the virus is waiting for the right time to resurrect. To find out if HIV was as old and as patient as this virus, scientists used state-of-the-art molecular clocks to calculate its age. They found that HIV is not an ancient virus. In fact, the evolutionary biologists at the University of Arizona who made the discovery described HIV as "surprisingly young."

Scientific discovery often involves wading through shit. To trace the origins of HIV, scientists had to squat in the depths of steamy central African forests and collect more than seven thousand piles of chimpanzee scat. Sifting through the poop, they found traces of a virus that looked a lot like HIV. It was the monkey version of the virus. They called it simian immunodeficiency virus "cpz," short for chimpanzee, or SIVcpz.

Back in the lab, they used a technique called molecular dating to trace the history of the virus. In the 1960s, scientists Linus Pauling and Emile Zuckerkandl came up with a hypothesis that would help researchers estimate the tick tock of the evolutionary clock and calculate the age of modern day viruses.

Biologist Motoo Kimura developed their work and found that DNA and protein sequences in different organisms evolve at nearly constant rates. That means you can analyze DNA and protein to figure out when one species diverged from another.

The story of HIV, the biggest pandemic to hit humankind, begins in 1492—give or take two hundred years—with a central chimpanzee (scientific name *Pan troglodytes troglodytes*) living in south-central Cameroon. This chimpanzee, let's call it chimp zero, lived in a region of the rainforest sandwiched between the Congo, Sanaga, and Ubangi rivers. One day, chimp zero went hunting.

Chimpanzees, which are not monkeys but apes, hunt small monkeys. Chimp zero ate two monkeys, a red-capped mangabey and a great spot-nosed monkey. Unbeknownst to chimp zero, both its appetizer and entree carried different strains of SIV.

Much like its human cousin, SIV spreads through blood and sex and also through bites. There are more than forty strains of the virus infecting apes and monkeys. The oldest strains have been around for thirty thousand years. The prevalence of SIV ranges from 50 percent in some species to 1 percent in others.

Viruses like Ebola and Nipah readily jump from bats to humans. West Nile virus infects horses, birds, and humans. But most strains of SIV prefer to stick to one species of ape or monkey. There's SIVver, an infection of African green monkeys that causes a dead-end infection in baboons, meaning an infected baboon can't pass the virus on to another animal.

There's SIVgor, which infects gorillas; SIVsmm, which infects sooty mangabeys; and then there are SIVgsn and SIVrcm, which infect the great spot-nosed monkey and the red-capped mangabey, respectively.

There's even an SIV strain that humans helped create by keeping primates in labs next to monkeys they would not have otherwise met. SIVmac infects laboratory macaques and is a result of scientists injecting macaques with blood from sooty mangabeys, who they didn't realize were infected with SIVsmm.

Foraging in the Cameroonian forest, chimp zero didn't realize its dinner was infected with SIV, possibly because many species of monkey don't fall sick from the infection. This avirulence, as scientists call it, might occur because monkeys and SIV evolved together over thousands of years. Over time they learned to live with one another, sort of like buying ear plugs to adjust to a noisy neighbor or leaving notes near the sink for a messy roommate who lets the plates pile up. You make adjustments and learn to put up with one another.

Chimpanzees, on the other hand, do get sick from SIVcpz. Chimps carrying the virus can show signs of a monkey version of AIDS, perhaps because SIVcpz is newer than some monkey strains of SIV and so chimps haven't had a chance to coevolve and get to know their virus.

Female chimps infected with SIVcpz are less likely to give birth, and if they do, their babies are more likely to die as infants. The overall death rate is ten to sixteen times higher among chimps infected with SIVcpz.

Back in 1492, or thereabouts, the great spot-nosed monkey that chimp zero had for dinner was infected with SIVgsn. The red-capped mangabey it ate was infected with SIVrcm. Inside the furry body of chimp zero, these two strains of SIV recombined to create a novel strain of SIV called SIVcpz.

This new virus had the ability to jump species from chimp to human.

But for the next four hundred or so years, SIVcpz seems to have stayed within the chimpanzee population. Then, in 1908, give or take twenty years, a chimpanzee infected with SIVcpz came across a human in southeastern Cameroon. The chimp may have bitten the human; the human may have hunted the chimp.

This discovery was made by Dr. Michael Worobey and his team at the University of Arizona, who place the chimp and human meeting somewhere south of the river Sangha, which divides Cameroon into north and south, and close to the river Ngoko, which flows near the border of the Democratic Republic of the Congo.

Inside that possibly wounded human, SIVcpz mutated and became HIV, a virus that would spread to every outpost of the world infecting more than seventy million people and killing half of them.

It didn't have to be that way. The first person infected with the virus, patient zero, could have lived a celibate and solitary life. She could have traveled little, socialized rarely, and kept the infection to herself. HIV could have had a different story, one where it was contained in a remote corner of the world, maybe even dying out. That's not what happened.

Between patient zero's infection in the early 1900s and up until the late 1950s, not much happened with HIV. People in central Africa most certainly contracted the infection, fell sick, and died. Some even passed it on to their children and lovers. But the infection simmered at low levels, and there was no widespread outbreak.

Colonialism changed that. Belgian, British, German, and French rule in central Africa brought humans and infected monkeys closer together, according to some anthropologists. It's more likely that a series of events, not a singular incident, sparked the epidemic.

These events—a hungry chimp, a rapidly mutating virus, an unlucky human—were fueled by colonialism and European exploitation in West Africa and central Africa. Centuries of tradition, long-standing patterns of migration, and behaviors were disrupted and transformed.

In medicine, there are meetings about mistakes. Meetings about the patient whose right kidney was removed when the left was diseased, the patient who was stitched up on the operating table with a scalpel inside his belly.

Most health care systems are designed with fail-safes to protect patients. Perhaps a senior doctor has to sign off on a prescription of a particularly powerful medicine before a resident can inject it, or a nurse must write on an operating room whiteboard the precise number of swabs used during surgery so that none are left inside the patient's chest.

But sometimes the fail-safes fail and at hotwash meetings doctors and administrators gather to detail the mishaps. Each mistake is likened to a slice of Swiss cheese with a big fat hole in the middle. On its own, that one hole may be of no consequence, but line it up next to another holey piece of cheese, and another mistake and then another, and you have a block of cheese that has a hole going right through it. One mishap after another creating a cavity that lets a deadly mistake pass all the way through.

That's what happened with HIV. Looking back at its origins like a detective trying to solve a murder mystery, there's the event in 1492, when chimpanzee zero ate two infected monkeys and brewed a new virus, SIVcpz, which had the potential to spread to humans. Then there's the event in 1908, when SIVcpz was transmitted to a human. And then there's nothing. Until 1959.

At this point in HIV's origin story, all roads lead back to the Congo. Or all railroads lead back there. In the late 1950s, as revolution brewed in the Belgian colony and riots exploded in its capital, Leopoldville, a person became infected with HIV. We don't know the person's name but we know his or her blood was swimming with the young virus, because a sample of it now sits in a laboratory in Tucson at the University of Arizona.

This sample is known in the medical literature as ZR59. It's the earliest sample of HIV. In Tucson, it shares a shelf with a piece of lymph node taken from a woman in 1960. The lymph node biopsy, labeled DRC60, is the second earliest sample containing HIV. It, too, was taken from a person in what was then Leopoldville in the Congo, now known as Kinshasa in the Democratic Republic of the Congo.

A few years before those samples were taken, HIV probably hopped onto a boat in Cameroon, sailed the river Sangha, and hopped off in the Congo. At the time, Congo's capital was one of the most connected cities in Africa. French and German colonial companies exploiting Cameroon for its rich reserves of ivory and rubber used the rivers and railroads to transport goods from Cameroon to Leopoldville.

Colonialism fueled the spread of HIV in a number of ways. It put Africans in closer proximity to apes infected with SIVcpz. Counter to the stereotypes, not all communities living in central Africa hunt monkeys and apes for food or skin. Some ethnic groups expressly prohibited the eating of ape meat, while others favored gorilla meat over chimpanzee. Colonization transformed these traditional practices.

Between 1895 and 1910, French and German companies sold tens of thousands of guns to Cameroonians in exchange for ivory and rubber. Some anthropologists say this encouraged bushmeat or game hunting in communities where it had not been common.

Other European colonialists forced the locals into rubber collecting, which meant spending weeks away from home inside forests with little to eat besides bushmeat. In the 1920s and 1930s, French and Belgian colonialists forced locals to first lay and then upgrade railway tracks—those workers were given bushmeat to eat.

Food and hunting practices changed, and so did the demographics. Trading posts set up along the Sangha, Congo, and Oubanghui rivers by French and German troops and traders, fed small villages with a steady stream of new visitors who had sex with local women. Soldiers, merchants, and laborers passed through in massive numbers, and rates of sexually transmitted infections soared. These simmering infections included syphilis, which causes open sores in the hands and genitals, welcoming entry points for HIV to seep into the body.

Forced labor, gun sales, bushmeat, and syphilis—the exploitation of rubber and ivory made Leopoldville a hotbed of HIV. Scientists refer to the region as the cradle of the AIDS pandemic, but it was more like a springboard. A confluence of factors, slices of Swiss cheese stacked with the holes perfectly aligned, turned the region into the birthplace of a global pandemic. It was in Kinshasa that a local killer became a mass murderer.

HIV jumped from chimps to humans and spread between people for seventy years before we had any idea what was happening. Now, epidemiologists can look back and estimate that by 1960, more than two thousand people in central Africa were infected with HIV. Molecular dating shows the virus arrived in Brazzaville from Cameroon as early as 1937.

Around the time that Cameroon gained independence from France on January 1, 1960, rates of HIV nearly tripled. Central Africa became an open and welcoming destination for Francophone people from around the world. In the early part of the 1960s, a program relocated hundreds of Haitian teachers to the Democratic Republic of the Congo. When those teachers returned to Haiti, they took HIV with them.

From Haiti, HIV traveled to the United States, arriving by the mid-1960s. We know this because in 1969 in St. Louis, Missouri, a teenager named Robert Rayford died of AIDS. No one knew it back then, but his was the earliest confirmed case of HIV in the United States. The virus was staking its ground on a new continent, ready to detonate a global pandemic.

There is more than one HIV. The HIV we've been talking about so far, HIV without any hyphens or numbers attached, is HIV type 1, or HIV-1, which has four groups, M, N, O, and P. Each of these groups was birthed by a separate ape-to-human transmission event.

Group M stands for "major." This is the HIV you fear, the strain that has caused a global pandemic and spread to eighty million people. Group M was first to be discovered. It's the virus found in a person in Kinshasa in 1959 and in the lymph node biopsy of a woman in 1960—the earliest samples of HIV in human tissue.

Group O stands for "outlier." Discovered in 1990, group O is much less common than group M, making up fewer than 1 percent of global infections. Most of the people infected with group O live in Cameroon, Gabon, and a few neighboring countries.

Group N was discovered in 1998 and is even more rare than group O. Group M likely comes from that densely forested area flanked by the rivers Sangha, Boumba, and Ngoko in southeastern Cameroon, whereas group N likely comes from the Dja Forest in south-central Cameroon. Analysis of its genes show it may have been passed to a human from a gorilla infected with SIVgor. That virus, SIVgor, was likely born when a gorilla brawled with a chimp infected with SIVcpz.

Only a dozen or so people have ever been diagnosed with HIV group N. All of them lived in Cameroon. Group P is even more rare. It has been found in only one person, also in Cameroon.

We can divide the pandemic strain of HIV, HIV type 1, group M, into nine subtypes or clades. Labeled A through K, these clades differ in their amino acids and surface proteins. Clade C is responsible for half of all HIV infections in southern Africa, India, and the Horn of Africa. Clade B is responsible for only 12 percent of infections worldwide but attracts most of the attention and research funding because it is mostly found in Americans and Europeans.

Then there is an entirely different strain of HIV known as HIV type 2, or HIV-2, found in Portuguese-speaking parts of the world. HIV-2 has a different origin story. It passed from monkeys to humans with an SIV precursor but its journey begins in a different animal, a gray-furred monkey with streaks of white across its eyelids called the sooty mangabey.

In 1986, a French researcher at the Institut Pasteur named François Clavel and Harvard veterinarian Phyllis Kanki discovered HIV-2. The virus is a distant cousin of HIV-1. Evolutionary biologists say the virus jumped from a sooty mangabey infected with SIVsmm to humans somewhere around the 1940s in Guinea-Bissau, a West African country two thousand miles north of Cameroon.

This explains the Portuguese connection. During the mid-fifteenth century up until 1974, Guinea-Bissau was a Portuguese colony. Today, although HIV-2 is less contagious than HIV-1 and less likely to be transmitted from mother to baby during birth, it is found in southern India, Gibraltar, and parts of West Africa—all places where Portuguese colonialists settled. During the independence wars in Guinea-Bissau, which lasted from 1961 to 1974, rates of HIV-2 spiked and the virus was transported to Portugal inside the bodies of repatriates and Portuguese soldiers.

In the early 1980s there were whispers in the virology world that infection with HIV-2 protected a person against infection with HIV-1. The opposite turned out to be true. HIV-2 increases a person's vulnerability to infection with HIV-1, and it's possible, but rare, that a person can be infected with both types of the virus. Co-infection is becoming even more rare. HIV-1 continues to expand its reach in West Africa, and HIV-2 is being steadily replaced by its deadlier cousin.

Just when you think you've gotten to know HIV, it dons a fresh disguise. The virus mutates constantly, making it a blurry bullseye.

Each time a virus particle reproduces, it mutates, changing its appearance and behavior in subtle ways, as if wearing a hat and sunglasses to evade recognition and capture. Humans mutate too; that's how evolution occurs and how our backs became straighter and skulls grew larger. But

HIV evolves a million times faster. It evolves so rapidly that inside one person there might be a hundred variants of the virus. They are all HIV, but they are different enough that medications may not work equally well against all of them.

And this is a problem in the search for a vaccine to treat and prevent HIV because vaccines need stable targets. Look at the hassle we face each year with the flu vaccine, every flu season demanding a new flu shot. The flu virus also mutates from season to season, switching up the proteins on its surface. That's why scientists play a guessing game each spring to predict which three or four strains will attack in the winter. If they guess right, the flu vaccine they design will work. If they get it wrong, the vaccine will be useless.

The guessing game has a scientific basis. In the Northern Hemisphere, scientists will look to flu epidemics in the Southern Hemisphere, where winter occurs during their summer. By watching which strains cause illness in the south, they can predict which flu strains might travel north.

There is work underway at the National Institutes of Health in the United States and elsewhere to develop a longer-lasting flu vaccine, but it will require discovering which parts of the flu virus don't change as much.

It's the same with HIV. If we can figure out what early HIV looked like—the HIV that existed before we knew about a mysterious illness in gay men in San Francisco and New York—and if we can see which parts of that young HIV still linger in the modern version, then we can use those older, more stable parts of the virus as targets for a vaccine.

In the 1980s and 1990s, when Joep was a young doctor, studying the origins of the virus may have seemed an extravagant pastime afforded to those who didn't have to face sickly patients and sign a dozen death certificates at the end of every night shift.

But unraveling the ropes of human history, untangling the tales of hunters, chimps, sailors, and scientists, shows how we are connected, vulnerable, and strong. Tracing HIV to its beginnings in a damp forest could help us overcome the virus. Origin stories could save humanity.

3 *The Epidemic*

Before the living dead roamed the hospital, the sharp angles of their bones poking through paper-thin bed sheets and diaphanous nightgowns, there was one patient, a harbinger of what would consume the rest of Joep's life.

Noah walked into the hospital on the last Sunday in November of 1981. It was Joep's sixth month as a doctor and a quiet day in the emergency room at the Wilhelmina hospital, a red brick building surrounded by gardens in the center of Amsterdam.

Noah was forty-two years old, feverish, and pale. His skin dripped a cold sweat. The insides of his cheeks were fuzzy with thick streaks of white fungus. And then there was the diarrhea. Relentless, bloody diarrhea. Noah's stomach cramped, his sides ached, he couldn't swallow food.

Doctors admitted him to the infectious disease ward, a former army barracks in the ninety-year-old hospital, where they puzzled over the streaky plaques of *Candida albicans*, a yeasty fungus growing inside his mouth, and the bacteria *Shigella* breeding inside his gut.

Noah swallowed spoonfuls of antifungal medicine. Antibiotics were pushed through his veins until his mouth turned a rosy pink and his bowels quieted. Still, the doctors were baffled by his unlikely conglomeration of symptoms. "The patient needs further evaluation," they wrote in his medical records. "He has anemia. And if the oral *Candida* recurs, it would be useful to check his immune function." They discharged him on Friday, December 11, 1981.

Had they read the *New England Journal of Medicine* on Thursday, December 10, they would have found nineteen Noahs in its pages.

Reports were coming in from Los Angeles and New York City of gay men dying from bizarre infections usually seen in transplant patients and rarely in the elderly. Like Noah, their immune systems had been annihilated and they were plagued with a dozen different bugs—ubiquitous microbes that rarely caused sickness in young men.

The week that Noah walked out of Wilhelmina hospital, the *New England Journal of Medicine* dedicated its entire "original research" section to articles on this strange plague. In one report, scientists from Los Angeles described four gay men who were brewing a fungus, *Pneumocystis carinii*, inside their lungs, and *Candida* inside their mouths and rectums. Doctors in New York City puzzled over fifteen men with worn-out immune systems and persistent herpes sores around their anus.

By the time the *New England Journal of Medicine* article was printed, only seven of the nineteen men in its pages were still alive.

The first hint of catastrophe arrived earlier that summer, just weeks after Joep graduated medical school. He had read the initial case reports in the June 5 issue of the *Morbidity and Mortality Weekly Report*, a bulletin from the US Centers for Disease Control.

Five short paragraphs told the story of five gay men. Each of them arriving at hospitals in Los Angeles with *Pneumocystis carinii* growing inside their chests.

The youngest man was twenty-nine years old. He had been diagnosed with the lung disease in February that year, around the same time that Joep was preparing for his final exams. By March, he was dead. An autopsy found his lungs riddled with foamy gray mold, white cysts, and patches of black where a second infection with cytomegalovirus transformed his lungs into thick slabs of rubbery tissue.

Two of the men were aged thirty; both were still alive but suffering fevers that had persisted for months. Like the others, they grew layers of white *Candida* on their tongues and inside their gullets. All the men were infected with cytomegalovirus—it had infiltrated their bladders, lungs, and rectums.

The oldest man was thirty-six years old. Cytomegalovirus lurked inside his eyeballs so that when doctors looked into his eyes they found the retina splotched with blood and dead tissue—an image their medical textbooks described as cheese and tomato pizza or scrambled eggs with ketchup.

The fifth man in the CDC case series was thirty-three years old. He was given medicines for the fungus in his lungs and the cytomegalovirus invading his body. He died in May of 1981.

Two weeks after the case series was published, Joep read a second round of case reports in the *Morbidity and Mortality Weekly Report*. This time nearly two dozen gay men in California were found with *Pneumocystis carinii* inside their lungs and a rare cancer beneath their skin.

The cancer was Kaposi's sarcoma and it wasn't new; it was discovered in 1872 by the Hungarian dermatologist Dr. Moritz Kaposi, but the cancer was usually seen in elderly Mediterranean men. It was caused by herpesvirus-eight, which invaded the cells lining the blood vessels sparking malignant tumors. Blood vessels would fragment and leak red cells, causing violaceous patches to grow beneath the skin.

Kaposi's sarcoma usually appeared on the shins and calves and then spread to the soles of the feet. Now it was cropping up on the cheeks and temples of young men. In some of those men, the cancer was indolent, sticking to skin or gums. In others, it was a fulminant disease attacking from the inside and sprouting lesions on their brains and bones. Most American doctors had never seen Kaposi's sarcoma.

In elderly Mediterranean men, the cancer grew slowly, so the men died with Kaposi's sarcoma—not from it. But as Joep flicked through the pages of the journal, he discovered that most of the men in the American report had died within months of looking in the mirror and seeing the first splotches of Kaposi's sarcoma on their faces.

The day after he read the bulletin, the news jumped from his medical journals to the front pages of the daily newspapers. "Rare Cancer Seen in 41 Homosexuals," the *New York Times* headline read. The article cited doctors who said they expected to see cases in cities around Canada, the United States, and even Europe.

Besides the cancer and lung infections, the men were diagnosed with parasitic infections such as giardia, and amoeba, and viruses like hepatitis B. Their immune systems were malfunctioning so that ubiquitous and usually benign infections were causing death. T cells and B cells had mysteriously vanished, and doctors couldn't understand why.

A *New York Times* article mentioned LSD and amyl nitrates—drugs swallowed and sniffed by some gay men to intensify orgasms. Could a tainted batch of poppers, the street name for the glass vials of amyl nitrate, have caused immune system dysfunction, leaving the men vulnerable to a slew of illnesses?

One doctor told the newspaper there was no danger to gay men and no sign of a plague. "The best evidence against contagion is that no cases have been reported to date outside the homosexual community or in women," he said.

The CDC wasn't so sure. It dispatched a group of Epidemic Intelligence Service officers to San Francisco. The disease detectives set up base in a downtown hotel, visited the city's bathhouses and scoured the sex clubs. They began interviewing gay men and brainstorming hypotheses about how the disease was spread.

Was it airborne like the measles or spread through inanimate objects, like conjunctivitis? Did it jump from person to person, or were all the sick men exposed to the same toxin? There were early comparisons between the new outbreak and hepatitis B, a virus spread through blood and sex, leaving some of the medical sleuths convinced they were facing a viral epidemic that was sexually transmitted.

Many of the sick were infected with cytomegalovirus, an infection that can temporarily quiet the immune system. In one of the journal articles, Dr. Michael Gottlieb suggested that cytomegalovirus could be a potential cause of the syndrome, but the journal editors wondered why more men weren't falling sick, since according to some studies, nine out of ten gay men had a history of infection with cytomegalovirus.

"What do young Africans, elderly Americans, renal-transplant recipients, and homosexual men have in common?" the editors asked. They offered more questions than they did answers. What was certain was that the nameless syndrome was not confined to the coastal United States. It was fanning across the country and possibly the world.

While Joep was reading the case reports an ocean away, thousands of people were already infected. Neither they nor their doctors knew it.

Four days after Noah walked out of the Wilhelmina hospital, a young man walked into the emergency room at the Onze Lieve Vrouwe Gasthuis, or Our Lady Hospital, a ten-minute bike ride away in east Amsterdam.

Dr. Peter Reiss was on call that Tuesday night, his long white coat flapping around his knees as he hurried from bed to bed. Peter and Joep had met in medical school, where they realized they were born a day apart. Joep was one day older than Peter, and he liked to remind his friend of this fact.

Peter picked up the new patient's chart and stroked his trim brown beard as he read the intake sheet. His bright blue eyes scanned the notes just as he had read the *New England Journal of Medicine* the previous Thursday.

He walked over to the cubicle and pushed aside the curtain. There was Daniel, a skinny nineteen-year-old with mousey blonde hair, sitting at the edge of the examination table. His skin was pale with bluish half-moons setting beneath his eyes. He was drenched in sweat and hacking a dry cough.

Daniel looked barely pubescent, Peter thought, and he checked the chart for his date of birth. There it was, February 1962. Daniel watched as his young doctor slipped blue gloves over his steady hands. Peter had a broad, reassuring smile and a calm manner.

"Tell me, how long have you been feeling sick?" he asked gently. Daniel had been ill since November. First, a prickly red rash dotted his chest and arms, then itchy red scabs appeared on his bottom. The diarrhea started soon after and he was running to the toilet every few hours. He had a fever that kept creeping higher.

Peter asked if he could palpate his neck and Daniel nodded. Pressing his fingers under the angles of his jaw, the pads of Peter's fingers found shotty lymph nodes as large as jelly beans. Peering inside Daniel's mouth, he saw a white blanket of *Candida* coating his tongue and tonsils. When he stepped back, Daniel coughed and caught his breath and Peter realized that the air had escaped his own lungs, too.

A teenaged boy with enlarged glands, oral thrush, and perianal herpes sounded a lot like the journal articles he had read on Thursday. The case reports flashed through his head: young gay men, history of drug use, American cities.

"Are you sexually active?" Peter asked softly.

Daniel looked away. "Yes," he whispered. "I had sex with a man for the first time ten weeks ago. He was much older than me, forty-two years old, I think. I heard he's very sick."

In the summer of 1981, the streets of Amsterdam's gay quarters thrummed with disco music and laughter. On Tuesday nights, self-proclaimed pretty boys gathered at the April bar on Reguliersdwarsstraat, their dark blue Valentino jeans hugging soft, perfumed skin. They pressed their bodies into one another, closed their eyes, and swayed beneath the neon lights.

Those seeking lubricious pleasures descended the stairs at the Viking bar, a few doors down, where nameless men roamed a pitch-black room and explored one another with fists and tongues.

A ten-minute walk away, leather daddies swigged beer at the Argos bar. Thick metal chains hung from the ceiling and a bull's head donated by a local butcher watched from the wall. At the Eagle bar across the street, men from the country's outermost islands hooked up with boys from the deep south, their chaps and harnesses squeaking at the bar.

Amsterdam was a safe haven. Lovers from the provinces could walk down the street and do the unthinkable: hold hands, hug, plant playful kisses on their boyfriend's faces. Here, there was safety in numbers— freedom in a place where gay men were met with smiles instead of slurs.

Those who took vacations in the United States reported back that Amsterdam was a lot like San Francisco with its kink bars and bathhouses, places where gay men could hang out and enjoy anonymous sex.

In both cities, the new illness was preying on love and freedom. If colonialism had sparked the spread of HIV from chimpanzees to humans, homophobia was the fuel that helped the epidemic spread from one person to another. The virus was exploiting the need for comfort and community as it swept through bedrooms and bathhouses in the Castro and on Reguliersdwarsstraat.

More than twenty bathhouses dotted San Francisco, including the Fairoaks Hotel, a converted apartment building on the corner of Oak and Stiner. Yoga classes ran alongside therapy sessions and group sex. Wooden-framed signs at the front desk advertised poppers and t-shirts at five dollars apiece.

Disease detectives from the CDC descended on these refuges to collect samples and stories, a nameless disease with an unknown mode of transmission giving them license to inject themselves into the private lives of strangers. They offered no answers, only long lists of questions: How many men did you have sex with? What kind of sex was it? Can you write down all your lovers' names?

The men offered up memories and saliva samples, fearful of what the government doctors would find inside their specimens. The disease detectives were trying to work the investigation like any other outbreak, following the same steps in their usual logical manner. Except this time, the world was watching and waiting for answers.

A handful of diseases have been eliminated from a few pockets of the globe, their numbers dwindling to levels that give humans a sense of dominance over the microbial world. But only one infectious disease has been eradicated: smallpox.

The mastermind behind the global erasure of that virus was Dr. Bill Foege, a looming figure who worked tirelessly to eradicate smallpox in the 1970s. In 1977, he was appointed director of the CDC by President Jimmy Carter.

But a few years into his tenure, Bill's scientific acumen was up against political fatuity. Carter lost the election to Ronald Reagan, who was supported by a political-action group called the Moral Majority. "AIDS is the wrath of God upon homosexuals," said its leader, Reverend Jerry Falwell.

Pat Buchanan, Reagan's communication director, said the illness was "nature's revenge on gay men."

Reagan said nothing. He uttered the word "AIDS" publicly for the first time in May of 1987 as he neared the end of his presidency. By that time, fifty thousand people were infected around the world and more than twenty thousand Americans had died.

To make matters worse, the Reagan administration demanded cuts in public health spending. Bill had to tighten his purse strings just as the biggest epidemic to hit humanity was taking off.

Even within the CDC, some leaders were doling out politically motivated advice. "Look pretty and do as little as possible," said Dr. John Bennett, assistant director of the division of the Center for Infectious Diseases. He was speaking to Dr. Don Francis, a young and outspoken epidemiologist who had returned from investigating the world's first outbreak of Ebola in Zaire.

Bill possessed a stronger will. Armed with political savvy and epidemiologic expertise, he instructed Dr. James Curran to assemble a team. James was head of the research branch of the CDC's Venereal Disease Control Division. By assigning him a new role, Bill was working the system to give James enough latitude to conduct what would be the most important investigation of their lives.

James gathered thirty Epidemic Intelligence Service officers and CDC staff to form a task force. Joined by Dr. Wayne Shandera, the Epidemic Intelligence Service officer assigned to Los Angeles County, the task force for Kaposi's sarcoma and Opportunistic Infections got to work.

The first item on the to do list in any outbreak investigation—even one as devastating as AIDS—is to come up with a case definition, a short list of criteria that will help other doctors look for cases. The disease detectives huddled around a table in their Atlanta headquarters and listed the major scourges of the new syndrome.

A case was defined as a person who had Kaposi's sarcoma or a proven opportunistic infection such as *Pneumocystis carinii* pneumonia. They had to be aged younger than sixty, and they couldn't have any underlying illness such as cancer or be on any medications that would suppress their immune system.

They shared the case definition with doctors around the country and by the end of 1981, as Noah and Daniel were walking into hospitals in Amsterdam, the CDC had a list of one hundred and fifty-eight American men and one woman who fit the description. Half of them had Kaposi's sarcoma, 40 percent had *Pneumocystis carinii* pneumonia, and one in ten had both. Looking back, the earliest case they could find was a man who fell sick in 1978.

They looked for connections between the cases and found themselves writing names on a blackboard and drawing white lines between the people who had sex with one another. A spider's web of a vast sexual network emerged. Thirteen of the nineteen men who were sick in southern California had had sex with the same man.

Task force Drs. David Auerbach and William Darrow cast their net wider, looking at ninety gay men across a dozen cities who fit the case definition. Forty of those men had sex with the same man, who was also sick.

Still, some were vehemently opposed to the idea that the syndrome was sexually transmitted. If it was spread through sex, why hadn't this happened before? But then came the summer of 1982 and reports of babies and hemophiliacs with *Pneumocystis carinii*. The common link was blood transfusions. This added a new mode of transmission. Like hepatitis B, the new illness was spread through sex and blood.

The CDC announced four groups of people were most vulnerable to the new illness, hemophiliacs, homosexuals, heroin users, and Haitians, and the disease earned a new name: 4H. With that public health announcement came public outrage and vitriol against those groups, especially gay men and Haitians. Houses were burned, children expelled from school, families forced to move towns because they were sick. Politicians sat complicit in their silence.

It was unparalleled, this confluence of public health, politics, clinical medicine, and public anxiety. The unknown disease was spreading faster than imagined. Humanity had never seen anything like it.

On a seemingly ordinary night shift in his first months as a doctor, Peter Reiss had tended to the first known Dutch person to be suffering acute HIV infection. Daniel, the nineteen-year-old in the emergency room, had been recently infected with HIV. His damp skin and sore throat evidence that the virus was multiplying at lightning speed inside him.

Peter's suspicions were accurate—Daniel did belong in the medical journals next to the case reports of sick men in San Francisco and Los Angeles—but it would be another year before Peter could prove his epidemiological hunch.

And four days before that night shift, Joep had wandered the corridors of the nearby Wilhelmina hospital while Noah, the first Dutch AIDS patient, was discharged from the ward, he and his doctors oblivious to the infection festering inside him.

In the spring of their medical careers, Joep and Peter had collided with two harbingers, but the pair did not realize they were teetering on the precipice of a global pandemic. It was as if the case reports from the medical journals had walked off the page and into their clinics dripping ink and leaking T cells along the hallways.

Clinical curiosity turned to horror as the wards began to fill with men, some their age, some even younger. Their cheeks were hollow, sunken eyes wide with horror, their temples and hands dotted with the stigmata of a nameless disease.

There was nothing the doctors could do to save them except to treat the shrewd infections feeding on their defenseless bodies. It was like playing whack-a-mole against two dozen opportunistic microbes. For *Pneumocystis carinii* pneumonia and *Candida*, they used antibiotics and antifungals. For the men tensing and collapsing, their bodies seizing under the weight of swollen, cyst-filled brains, they used antiparasitic medicines.

But for herpes, cytomegalovirus, and Kaposi's sarcoma, they had little to offer except morphine. Eventually, to treat Kaposi's sarcoma, they would irradiate the men and inject chemicals into each lesion.

Forty kilograms, thirty kilograms, the men withered down to their skeletons and sat, expressionless, catatonic. Trying to make flesh stick to their bones became an obsession. Within six to seven weeks, some developed dementia as their peers watched in horror. Is that going to happen to me? they asked the doctors. Will I forget my name?

And then there was the diarrhea—inexorable, bloody diarrhea, profuse and humiliating. The patients stewed in their own excrement until nurses lifted them out of the mess. Their skin, sodden and stinking, disintegrated into open sores. One young man in the corner of Joep's ward suffered diarrhea for a year before he died.

Joep turned for guidance to Dr. Sven Danner, an internal medicine consultant ten years his senior. Sven was a tall, no-nonsense man, who adored teaching as much as he enjoyed the detective work of diagnosing patients. Like Joep, he was ambitious, curious, and driven.

When Sven saw manifestations of the new illness on his patients' skin and in their brains, lungs, and bellies, he assembled a team of the hospital's best dermatologists, neurologists, pulmonologists, and gastrointestinal doctors. If the syndrome attacked each organ, they would fight back, defending each system as best they could.

Joep bombarded Sven with questions, and Sven turned to the medical literature for answers. They relished this fresh challenge as much as they resented it. Sven had deliberately stayed away from oncology because the palliation and suffering were too depressing, and here he was, dishing out morphine and impotent antibiotics.

There were moments of bizarre wonder. Bewildered by the volume of diarrhea their patients were producing and confused about what was causing it, they hunkered down with textbooks and sent multiple stool samples to the microbiology lab.

In some of their patients' guts, they found the bacteria *Shigella*, but in others a hodgepodge of bugs had taken up residence, including a parasite called *Isospora belli*. Sven scratched his head; he had never received a report from the microbiology lab quite like this one. When he searched the literature for advice on how to treat *Isospora*, he found answers—in a veterinary journal.

"So how much antibiotic do I give him?" asked a bemused Joep.

"It says here how much to give a cow," said Sven, pointing to a veterinary article and wrinkling his brow. He picked up a pen. "Let's calculate what dose to give a human."

They tried out new medicines, tinkered with dosages of old ones, and tried to combine clinical acumen with clinical dexterity. But there were times when they felt useless.

Years spent poring over pharmacology textbooks amounted to blank prescription pads, empty hands, lowered heads, and condolences. Desperate to make his patients feel better, Joep found himself doling out words of encouragement and empathy.

Medicine was forced back to basics. Gone was any reliance on diagnostics—they couldn't test their way out of this conundrum. With science frantically playing catch-up to a syndrome that had outfoxed it, they resorted to the Hippocratic techniques of observing and listening to the anxious despair of their charges. "I don't know" and "We are trying everything" were phrases that peppered Joep's bedside speech, and he hated it. He had questions, too.

Like how had he become an expert in palliative care? Unknowingly, unwillingly, he was becoming skilled at adjusting the dose of morphine drips, fluffing and positioning pillows to cushion hip bones jutting through skin, prescribing the perfect dose of diarrhea medicine—anything to ease the pain and indignity of death.

Some days they invited death onto the ward. The requests came from the men who were exhausted, emaciated, petrified. Won't you just help me end it? Don't I deserve repose? And so they found themselves huddled in corners, conferring with their patients' lovers about a moral gray zone and the logistics of dying.

The patients wanted farewell parties, where they would flick through photo albums with friends and reminisce on the good times, the pain-free times. Champagne corks were popped as friends gathered around the hospital bed. They sang songs and whispered goodbyes, and one of the doctors would hang a glass bottle of saline from a metal frame and slowly switch the salt water for a lethal dose of pentobarbital.

Physician-assisted suicide was not new in Holland in the 1980s, it was practiced there and in other parts of the world, but in the Dutch tradition of speaking openly, even about morally ambiguous topics, euthanasia had been discussed in the courts. There were guidelines to help doctors navigate the tortuous territory: consult with the patient on at least four separate occasions, make sure they are competent, meet with their family physician, speak to their loved ones, only consider their request if medicine cannot alleviate their suffering.

The doctors knew the guidelines; they had studied them in medical school, but they never anticipated confronting thorny end-of-life issues at the very start of their careers.

A few carried out a dozen or so farewell parties, sometimes choosing to mix pancuronium bromide with pentobarbital so there would be no jerking in the patient's final moments, only soft sighs as flaccid muscles relaxed into a perpetual slumber. It was not the pharmacology they expected to use, but they felt it was their one helpful contribution.

Joep was halfway into his case presentation during a grand rounds lecture one morning when a poem appeared on the slide projector behind him. "Oops," he said, with a smirk. "How did that get there?"

In the audience were a hundred senior medical faculty, residents, and students. They shuffled in their seats and fiddled with the rubber loops of their stethoscopes, their eyes scanned the poetic couplets searching for a clue about white cells or fevers.

In the back row, the chief of medicine, Hans Sauerwein, took a folded piece of paper from his white jacket and dropped it into the pocket of the internal medicine resident sitting next to him. The plan had been carefully devised. The chief was to deposit the gift—a printed copy of the entire poem—right at the moment when Joep pretended to have mixed up his grand rounds presentation, displaying the poetic stanza instead of a table of bloodwork results.

Never mind that the meeting was attended by the stuffiest chiefs of medicine and earnest medical students looking to score points—Joep had important work to do. He was seducing his latest object of desire.

He employed one of the more laid-back chiefs of medicine, Hans, to place the printed copy of the poem into the girl's pocket hoping she would later realize that the very public courting ritual was staged entirely for her benefit.

Hans thought the whole affair foolish but amusing. Joep would fall for another woman the next month, and Hans would probably play along in that game, too. It broke up the tedium of the long case presentations and the never-ending ward rounds. Joep's romantic pursuits reminded him of the hormones rushing through the veins they pricked each day, the beating hearts that lay beneath the chests they examined.

There were times during his internship when Joep became a recluse. Lectures and labs flew by while he lay sprawled across the sofa in his east Amsterdam flat, his arched eyebrows rising and falling with each turn of the page. He was learning medicine from Charles Bovary, the French doctor with a passion for dominoes and public houses. No matter that Joep's literary muse skipped medical school classes to learn how to mix cocktails and make love.

Bovary was a bad influence. He crammed for exams and almost flunked the first set of tests. Joep was far more diligent and academically astute, but he was consumed by the doctor's drama, parental interference, and marital strife. If medicine was about saving lives, literature was about living a life worth saving.

He pined for the drama he discovered in the tomes of European literature he finished faster than a bottle of his favorite red wine, the alcohol turning stale in his glass as he fell deeper and deeper into the plot twists.

Joep liked to reread his favorite book, Elias Canetti's *Auto-da-Fe*, named after the public burning of heretics during the Spanish Inquisition. The protagonist was Doktor Peter, a scholarly recluse who revered books more than life itself. He lived only to enjoy his great library of classical literature. Doktor Peter's life was comically overturned by his marriage to Therese, his illiterate housekeeper, with whom he had little in common.

Joep's nonfictitious medical role model was Jan Jacob Slauerhoff, Holland's most famous poet and novelist, whom he talked about as a young boy with his sister. The asthmatic writer compiled poems while studying medicine at the University of Amsterdam in the early 1900s. Slauerhoff published his first poem in a communist magazine and later edited the student newspaper, *Propria Cures*. Many considered him a *poète maudit*, a poet living life on the borders of society. His romantic, unfinished style of poetry dwelled on loneliness and the longing for love and home.

Nowhere but in my poems can I dwell
Nowhere else could I a shelter find.

He was a bohemian medical student. His nonconventional and confrontational style earned him dozens of enemies across the country, so that when Slauerhoff graduated from medical school he found it difficult to land a job in the Netherlands. He became a ship's doctor instead, working for the Dutch East Indies Company and writing novels along shipping routes. He became a global voyager sailing to Asia and Africa and eventually setting up his own clinic in Tangiers.

Joep imagined himself as Dr. Yuri Zhivago, a sensitive poet-physician who auscultated hearts while composing couplets in his head. The Russian doctor was the embodiment of empathy and idealism in a world of war and religious revolution. In art, Yuri found not only solace but a meaning for life.

Both Yuri and Joep buried their parents too young and both struggled to heal that wound through public service. They grappled with injustice and religion, and both doctors hurt the women they loved by falling in love with the women who worked alongside them.

Joep had a habit of proposing marriage to every woman he fell in love with—and there were many. First there was Marian, a medical student. He proposed to her while he was still in medical school, still toying with the idea of becoming a writer.

He suggested they get married during a trip to New York City and was surprised when she said yes. Some women dismissed his playful proposals, rolling their eyes at the hopeless romantic who sulked when they turned him down.

They didn't consider him conventionally handsome. His nose was a little crooked, his teeth were less than straight. But when his lips stretched from a smirk into a wide-mouthed smile, they were enamored.

He had a girlfriend when he met the tall nurse with the wavy brown hair down to her elbows. There was an ethereal quality about her, as if she could whisk him away to a land where there were no rules.

Joep first spotted Heleen Stok in the hospital on New Year's Eve. He walked up to her on the ward and said, "I'm going to marry you." She looked him up and down, taking in the puckish grin, the shirt with the collar unbuttoned. It was a moment of daring from an often shy man.

Heleen came from an upper middle-class family in Amsterdam. Her parents owned a home in the Vondelpark neighborhood, and it was in that leafy urban playground that they took their first double dates, Heleen and Joep holding hands next to Karel Koch and his girlfriend, Henriette Scherpbier, a pediatric resident.

Karel was a year younger than Joep and still in medical school. They met on the wards, where Joep was his supervisor, and in between conversations about platelets and chest X-rays, they had animated discussions about Joan Didion's memoirs, V. S. Naipaul's prose, and the merits of Nabokov's *Lolita*. "I have a great supervisor!" Karel said to Henriette when he arrived home from the hospital one evening. "You've got to meet him!"

"Jooopy!" Heleen called to her beau as the pair wandered through the park toward the bandstand. She was the only person to ever give him a nickname. He held her close as they lay on the grass, letting the sun and guitar chords wash over them.

He loved music, but he wasn't musically gifted. Karel, on the other hand, played clarinet, sang in a band, and attended music conservatory for two years before medical school. Joep was a little jealous of Karel's artistic talents and, unable to hold his tongue, told him so. Karel shrugged it off. Joep regularly turned up at his gigs and danced enthusiastically to the band's songs.

One evening, they drove from Amsterdam to Utrecht to watch Karel's band perform, then they drove ten hours through the night to Chatel, a town in the French Alps, for a skiing holiday. They stopped in Heerlen to pay a quick visit to Joep's mother.

Weaving through the winding mountain roads across Switzerland and into France, Joep clutched the steering wheel with his long fingers until his knuckles turned white. Snow flurries fell on the windscreen. Joep turned the windscreen wipers to their most frantic setting.

"I need to pull over!" he yelled.

"But you can't stop here! We've got to keep going!" said Karel.

The tires careened on ice and Joep gripped the wheel tighter. He wanted to strap snow chains over the tires, but there was nowhere safe to pull over on the narrow mountain road. He looked out of the window and down the precipitous drop to his left. His heart was pounding. He kept his eyes on the road and his ears on Karel.

They arrived at the alpine village and settled into a cabin, emptying the car of beer, food, and stacks of books which Joep had stuffed into the trunk. Karel, Henriette, and Heleen sat back with beer and looked out at the vista, a stunning horizon of white powder and snowcapped peaks. Joep's head was buried in a book about genetics. A pile of novels sat on the floor beside him.

The next morning, they crossed the border into Switzerland to hit the slopes. "God verdomme!" said Joep, tumbling down the mountain, his legs flailing. Heleen threw her head back and laughed before whizzing down the slope to rescue her boyfriend, who had collapsed in a pile of broken skis and snow.

On New Year's Eve of 1981, Noah felt feverish. Three weeks after walking out of the Wilhelmina hospital, he shuffled back in. His pulse was slowing, his temperature was spiking. *Candida* coated his tongue, *Shigella* grew in his gut. Doctors performed a colonoscopy, treated him with antifungals and antibiotics, and discharged him on New Year's Day.

By April of 1982, purple splotches spread over his face and chest and he felt short of breath. He went to a newly opened hospital, the Academic Medical Centre, in east Amsterdam, where Joep was now working.

"The clinical picture is compatible with what has been described in the literature as Gay Immunocompromised Syndrome," doctors there wrote. "The patient has no cellular immunity." They treated the infections and performed biopsies of his lungs. When Noah's kidneys failed, they put him on dialysis, but it was too late. Noah went into septic shock and died on May 1, 1982.

Less than a year into the epidemic, Joep was growing weary of the death certificates, the quotidian duties of clinical medicine, of patching up broken skin and plying puckered mouths with medicine only for another opportunistic infection to arrive and undo his hard work. The disease was winning. It would not be conquered on the ward—there had to be a better way.

And then Jaap Goudsmit arrived. He was three years older than Joep, astute, witty, and sporting a constant twinkle in his eye. Jaap had left the Netherlands in 1978 as soon as he graduated medical school, eschewing his country's nascent virology training to study at the US National Institutes of Health. A young scientist needed to be surrounded by Nobel laureates, he said, and he found just that environment at the NIH.

Jaap and Joep met one morning after grand rounds as the crowd was trickling out of the lecture theater, doctors dissipating to every corner of the hospital. The pair lingered between rows of chairs, and Jaap told Joep that he was back in Amsterdam to study for a PhD with Dr. Jan van der Noordaa, one of the country's top scientists. They were going to set up a virology lab.

The discussion soon turned from viruses to literature, and they dared themselves to create a list of the top one hundred novels, jotting down titles by Chekhov and Tolstoy. Jaap hadn't read all the books that Joep was adding to the list, but he instinctively trusted his literary expertise.

Jaap was forming an alliance with Sven Danner, Joep's clinical mentor, as well as Drs. Roel Coutinho and Peter Schellekens. Peter worked at the Netherlands Blood Transfusion Service, and Roel was an epidemiologist at the Municipal Health Service of Amsterdam. He had recently returned from a stint in Senegal, where he worked in a thirty-bed hospital treating survivors of war from neighboring Guinea-Bissau. Back in the Netherlands, Roel had taken a job that nobody else wanted.

Infectious diseases were passé, they told him. Are you sure you want to be head of public health at the Municipal Health Service of Amsterdam? Roel was sure. He began to study the epidemiology of sexually transmitted diseases among the city's injecting drug users and gay men.

The men weren't too bothered about syphilis and gonorrhea, they told him. There were treatments for those. What really concerned them was hepatitis B, because the medicines were toxic and often useless.

Roel enrolled a few hundred gay men to test an experimental hepatitis B vaccine made from the plasma of people who were long-term carriers of the virus. The idea was to take chunks of the virus floating in the blood of those who were infected and use those pieces to bolster the immune system of people at risk of contracting hepatitis B. The injecting drug users were at risk, because they sometimes shared needles; the gay men were vulnerable to infection if they didn't use condoms.

The plasma of hepatitis B carriers came from the Blood Transfusion Service, where Peter worked. When the first cases of a new, perhaps sexually transmitted disease appeared in the journals, Peter and Roel realized they had a head start. They could use their large cohorts to study the new syndrome. The men they knew so well were some of the city's most vulnerable people when it came to the new syndrome.

There were mutterings that the syndrome might be caused by a virus, which prompted Roel to contact Jaap. They hatched a plan. They would use Roel's cohorts to study how the disease spread among gay men in Amsterdam. Sven was their direct link to patients on the ward, patients who were carrying in their blood massive amounts of the mystery pathogen, and Jaap would work on developing a test for the illness. They were joined by Frank Miedema, who worked at the Central Laboratory of the Blood Transfusion Service.

The Dutch quartet was born, and some likened them to a politburo. They collaborated with a passion and fought so fiercely that after their meetings Roel would lose his car. Utterly discombobulated, he wandered around unable to locate where he had parked it—he was still seeing red from the scientific dispute they had been embroiled in. The four men needed each other to progress their scientific work, but the fights about how to do the work got so bad that outside mediators had to be called in to keep them together.

"I did the study in my lab, so why should I put your name on my paper?" one would say.

"Well this sounds like the time you gave a presentation using half of my data and forgot to mention my name once," came the response.

One night when Frank told his wife about a meeting of the quartet, his wife said, "I wish you talked to me with such passion and intensity. It sounds like you're having a love affair."

The passion produced some of the most sophisticated discoveries about HIV, and the quartet would soon be written about in science journals and discussed at medical meetings, the phenomenal combination of clinician, virologist, epidemiologist, and hematologist. They would give the Americans a run for their money.

Joep wanted in on the affair. But first he needed to get his PhD. He joined van der Noordaa's lab in the spring of 1983 with the chief as his main supervisor and Jaap as second supervisor. He would switch between the ward and the lab, continuing to care for patients while running experiments on the fourth floor.

And he continued to scribble titles on the list of the top one hundred novels with Jaap. "I've just read *Now* by Turgenev and it needs to be added to the top one hundred," Joep said to Jaap one day. "Fine," said Jaap. "But that means another book has to be kicked off."

In literature, as in science, there was space for only so much talent.

4 *Learn Your Enemy*

The virology lab hummed with the sounds of centrifuges spinning tubes of infected blood, the chhttt chhttt of students spraying alcohol onto wooden benches, and the occasional shudder of the tall freezers that lined the freshly painted white walls.

Joep was pouring and pipetting four floors below the wards where his patients perished, where their lovers pleaded with him to save them. The lab offered respite from the confounding clinical syndrome he couldn't fully grasp, the questions he couldn't answer. Amid the microscopes, freezers, and test tubes, there was hope—a tingling feeling of anticipation that he and his colleagues were on the brink of discovering something big.

The virology lab at the University of Amsterdam's Academic Medical Center (AMC) was a state-of-the-art setup, a world away from the old lab in town, which had been housed in an eighteenth-century brick building. Here, the researchers were surrounded by large glass windows and a specially sealed area within the lab where they worked with highly contagious bodily fluids.

The lab was run by Jan van der Noordaa, whom the young scientists called the Grand Old Man or the Godfather of virology. Jaap Goudsmit was his second in command. It was a crowded, frantic place charged with big ideas and bigger egos. With growing interest in the new plague, Joep found that other doctors had piled their lab notebooks onto his desk in one of the ten offices and he was forced to share his desk.

They argued over space and whose name would be added to the list of authors for a particular paper. Once their name was added they fought over the order of their name in the list of authors, vying for first, second, or last author—other spots offered less prestige. Van der Noordaa monitored the tension from his office, which he didn't share with anyone. The Godfather of virology wasn't interested in having his name on papers, but he did want to keep the fighting among his scientists confined to the lab so that others wouldn't get a whiff of the tension.

While Joep was hunched over his microscope and fighting his own battles in Amsterdam, scientists in France and America were going head to head to find the virus that caused AIDS.

Epidemiologists had pieced together clues about who was infected and where. They had scribbled social networks charting who had sex with whom and figured out the infection was spread through blood and semen. They were almost certain the cause was a virus. Now the world's top virologists were getting involved, and things were about to get messy.

Dr. Robert Gallo, known to his colleagues as Bob, worked at the National Institutes of Health in Maryland in a lab close to the one where Jaap Goudsmit had trained. A few years before the AIDS epidemic began, Bob discovered the first retrovirus, a bug that works backward by turning its RNA into DNA.

Bob wasn't interested in AIDS. He was still working on retroviruses, and it wasn't clear that the cause of AIDS was that kind of virus. But Don Francis, the CDC disease detective who worked on the AIDS taskforce, was aggressive in pleading with Bob for help. We have very few resources at the CDC and there's no one who has your technical expertise, Don said.

Once Bob joined the race, there were problems. He was known for being difficult to work with, and when Don ran into difficulties he asked a colleague for advice.

"Treat him like a seven-year-old," she said.

"But we're adults," said Don, "and this is a very important epidemic."

Once he was in the race, the struggle to identify the cause of AIDS consumed Bob. That was his personality, some of his peers said. He was doggedly determined and hard to work with but one of the finest scientists in the world. It was his mission to beat the French scientists, and that drive is what led to one of the biggest scandals in the history of science.

Bob's French counterpart was Luc Montagnier at the Institut Pasteur in Paris. His team had lymph nodes from two gay Frenchmen nicknamed Bru and Lai, and they were trying to coax the virus out of their lymph nodes and into cell cultures. But with little information about the virus they were trying to extract, they were struggling. It was a disaster. If they couldn't grow the virus, they couldn't study it.

Then in early 1983, Luc and his colleagues, Françoise Barré-Sinoussi and Jean-Claude Chermann, managed to isolate the virus from Bru's lymph node. They named it JBB/LAV after Bru's initials and lymphadenopathy-associated virus. They published their results in the journal *Science* in May 1983.

They sent samples of the virus to Bob and his team, a common practice in science, where the aim is to prove your results by asking your peers to reproduce your experiments.

But there was a problem. Bob's team was already working with blood from infected Americans. They were also trying to coax the virus out of the samples and somehow—there are different theories about how this happened—their samples became contaminated with the virus from France.

A few months later, when Gallo announced he had discovered the cause of AIDS, what he had actually "discovered" was the virus that Luc's team had sent from Paris.

Gallo went ahead and gave his "new" virus a name. Since he had discovered the first human retroviruses—HTLV I and HTLV II—he named this virus HTLV III.

The French and American teams were supposed to be working together, and at the time apparently no one knew about the viral mix-up. Luc thought he had isolated the virus out of his sample and that Bob had isolated it from his own samples. They decided to make a joint announcement that both groups had found the cause of AIDS.

But the Reagan administration had a different plan. Deathly silent about AIDS for so long, it wanted to jump on this new, apparently American discovery, and in April 1984 the secretary of health and human services held a news conference. To a room full of reporters, Margaret Heckler declared that it was Bob who had discovered the virus that causes AIDS, and it was called HTLV III. Bob stood for applause.

The Dutch scientists watched with intrigue and wondered how this would play out. They were focused on their own experiments, mostly looking at how the body responded to infection with the mystery virus and how it caused their patients to suffer and die.

The rest of the world was watching, too. In Paris, Luc was furious. He responded to the American press conference with lawsuits, and US authorities began to investigate Bob, his team, and their experiments. The US Federal Office of Research Integrity found Bob and his colleague, Dr. Mikulas Popovic, guilty of scientific misconduct. But then a different investigation cleared Bob's name. The inquiries stretched out over years and across different government agencies. At one point the FBI was called in to investigate the investigation.

In one report investigators said that an early draft of Bob's paper included comments from Mikulas. He had written that the French virus was likely the cause of AIDS and that he was using it as his reference for the experiments. Bob had scribbled next to these sentences: "Mika, are you crazy?" and then scratched out the comments.

The investigators asked why Bob couldn't just give the French team credit for their discovery. His lawyer explained that Bob was too angry and too emotional.

The fight escalated until 1987, when Reagan invited French prime minister Jacques Chirac to the United States for his first official visit, so they could bury the disagreement between the two scientists.

Bob and Luc signed a seven-page document detailing the chronology of HIV's discovery, but they didn't reach a verdict on who first isolated the virus.

Then in March 1987, Reagan made an announcement from the Oval Office. "This agreement opens a new era in Franco-American cooperation, allowing France and the United States to join their efforts to control this terrible disease in the hopes of speeding the development of an AIDS vaccine or cure."

That was supposed to be the very public, very official end of the disagreement, but the festering rivalry would be reignited in the next century. In 2008, Luc and his colleague Françoise Barré-Sinoussi won the Nobel Prize in Physiology or Medicine for the discovery of HIV. Bob was not mentioned.

From its first time in a lab, HIV was revealing science's dirty side.

Look through a microscope and meet HIV. Some viruses are naked, but HIV greets you wearing a coat. Magnified two hundred thousand times the ball-shaped virus spins and twirls, revealing a coat studded with protein stalks. A trio of leaf-shaped proteins hangs from each stalk. These leaves are the virus's keys into your cells.

The leaves are dipped in a sugar that sweetly conceals them from detection by the immune system, a cunning and necessary ploy, because HIV preys on the very cells designed to kill it—T helper cells.

T helper cells are the ringleaders of the immune system. When an intruder breaches the body, T helper cells sound a chemical siren jolting their cousins, B cells and cytotoxic T cells, from their slumber.

On the surface of T helper cells are proteins called CD4 receptors. Other cells of the immune system use these receptors to introduce T helper cells to bugs invading the body. HIV needs no introduction. Swimming through veins and arteries, the virus seeks out the chemical scent of the CD4 receptors on T helper cells. It turns them into a door handle.

The sweet leaves flapping on HIV's coat latch onto the CD4 receptors and pull the T helper cell into a tight embrace. When it is firmly attached to the CD4 receptor, HIV pulls a second, smaller receptor into its embrace. The second is usually the CCR5 receptor, which juts out of the surface of the T cell, but sometimes HIV opts for a receptor called CXCR4.

HIV holds on to the T helper cell and refuses to let go. The viral life cycle has begun, and one HIV particle will spawn a billion more. No matter that HIV is dwarfed by the T helper cell, which stands three hundred and fifty times bigger than the virus.

Bound to the T cell, HIV sheds its coat and spills its guts into the cytoplasmic mush. Out pours the capsid, a bullet-shaped cocoon that houses HIV's genes and enzymes. The viral cocoon is built of fifteen hundred blocks of a protein known as p24.

The viral cocoon shatters inside the T helper cell, releasing two strands of viral RNA. They float into the cytoplasm, a round blob swaying near their tails. The RNA contains instructions for making HIV. The blob is the enzyme reverse transcriptase.

HIV works backward. Instead of DNA turning into RNA and making protein—the central dogma of biology—HIV uses the enzyme reverse transcriptase to turn viral RNA into DNA. The enzyme is quick, rebellious, and sloppy. As it converts RNA into DNA, reverse transcriptase makes mistakes and doesn't bother to proofread its work.

Some viruses, especially those that contain DNA instead of RNA, produce perfect clones of themselves. Not HIV. Because reverse transcriptase is clumsy, one particle of HIV can produce a hundred different variations of itself. That means a person infected with the virus can carry hundreds of HIVs inside them, each virus particle a distant relative of the next. This is one way that HIV evades the treatments designed to stop it.

With its RNA turned into DNA, HIV uses an enzyme called integrase to carry its DNA into the nucleus of the T helper cell. Integrase acts like a pair of molecular scissors. It snips the human DNA, inserts HIV's DNA, and glues the two together.

Now the virus sits back and lets the human cell do the work. The T helper cell's own machinery reads the human DNA as well as the viral DNA and turns them both into long strands of RNA. The T helper cells ribosomes—small protein factories that float in the cytoplasm—turn the RNA into the proteins needed to make new copies of HIV. The new proteins are cut to size by the viral enzyme protease. The naked virus particles gather and float to the surface of the T helper cell.

HIV hijacks the immune system and turns our safety net into a virus-making factory. Infected T helper cells churn out all the components needed to make new HIV particles. More p24 proteins are synthesized, more blobs of reverse transcriptase and integrase enzymes are made.

The T helper cell even makes the leaves that HIV will wear on its coat and use to attach to T helper cells. Where does that coat come from? On its way out of the human cell, HIV steals a piece of the T helper cell's membrane and makes itself a new jacket. HIV is a thief. It is a usurper of cellular machinery. HIV targets the cells we rely on to keep infections at bay and by commandeering T helper cells, HIV rules the immune system.

With no ringleader to rally them into war, B cells and cytotoxic T cells become useless. The body is left vulnerable to infection with a jumble of usually harmless bugs. HIV likes company. It empowers more bugs to join in its hostile takeover of the human body.

Joep relished competition. Leaving a lab technician to fiddle with pipettes and petri dishes, he scuttled between the lab and the ward, taking samples from patients and helping other students with their experiments while working on his own.

There was a tension around him. A feeling that time was compressed and there weren't enough hours in the day to poke and prod the virus from every angle and answer all his questions. Some mornings he pushed past the other students in the lab and shouted at those who got in his way. His sharp words could make his lab mates cry and when that happened, he would dash out of the hospital and return with a plastic bag full of books. He handed out paperbacks as peace offerings.

Most PhD virologists spend years studying minutiae—a three amino acid stretch in one corner of the virus or the tip of the leaf hanging off the virus's coat. Joep was not typical. He spent four years studying different parts of the virus, how it took over the immune system and how it caused disease.

He published eleven papers on AIDS in his first years as a PhD student; often two or three of his studies would appear side by side in the same issue of the *Lancet* or the *Journal of AIDS*, some of the most prestigious medical journals in the world.

He studied an antiparasitic drug called amprolium used in chickens and found it eased the incessant diarrhea of AIDS patients. With Peter Schellekens, Jan van der Noordaa, and Sven Danner he wrote a review of thirty-six Dutch AIDS patients, describing the bugs that had taken over their blood, brains, and intestines.

And then there was a paper he wrote in 1985 with Jaap and Peter Reiss. It was about a nineteen-year-old boy who became infected with AIDS a few weeks after he had sex with a man for the first time. It was Daniel, the young, sickly man whom Peter met on one of his very first night shifts as a doctor in 1981.

Less than four years after Daniel and Peter first met in the emergency room a test was developed for AIDS. It was called ELISA, short for enzyme-linked immunosorbent assay. The test didn't detect HIV in the blood. Instead, it looked for antibodies that the immune system made when confronted with the virus.

Antibodies are Y-shaped proteins that hunt for bugs. Some bugs are good at hiding from immune system cells, but antibodies can attach to them and flag them, letting cells like phagocytes swoop in and enjoy a meal. Antibodies can also activate a type of immune system cell weapon called the natural killer cell.

When it was announced that there was an antibody test for AIDS, Peter ran to the lab at the Onze Lieve Vrouwe Gasthuis and pulled Daniel's samples from the freezer. He had stored the blood in hopes of this very moment. He thawed the tubes labeled "December 18" and "December 28," ran them through the new test, and waited.

The first blood sample, taken three days after Daniel walked into the hospital, was negative. There were no antibodies to the virus in his blood that day. But the blood taken on December 28 was swimming with antibodies. Daniel's immune system had reacted to the virus and started to make antibodies while he was a patient in the hospital.

Peter's hunch had been accurate—the teenager did belong in the pages of the *New England Journal of Medicine* and the *Morbidity and Mortality Weekly Report* alongside the case reports of gay men in San Francisco and Los Angeles.

Peter had written a medical journal article about Daniel in 1983. Its title posed the question: Could this patient have a mild form of AIDS? But what Daniel was really suffering from was acute HIV infection. He had been infected with the virus probably only a few weeks before he walked into the OLVG hospital.

Doctors didn't know about acute HIV infection until March of 1985, when Dr. David Cooper, an Australian immunologist who diagnosed the first AIDS case in Australia, published a paper in the *Lancet*. It was titled "Acute AIDS Retrovirus Infection: Definition of a Clinical Illness Associated with Seroconversion." Peter had read the article and thought back to that night shift when he had first met Daniel.

It takes the immune system anywhere from a few weeks to a few months to make antibodies to HIV, a process that scientists call seroconversion. Daniel had seroconverted before Peter's eyes, Peter just didn't have a way to prove it back in 1981. There was no test for antibodies and not even a good understanding of which antibodies were made to fight the virus.

When Joep began work on his PhD in 1983, he studied the way these antibodies formed and evolved in response to HIV. The cohort of gay men that Roel Coutinho had been working with since the 1970s gave him a head start to make important discoveries.

He looked at the blood of fifteen men enrolled in Roel's hepatitis B vaccine trial and found that when they were infected with HIV, the first antibodies their immune system made were directed against HIV's p24 protein, the building block that forms the virus's inner cocoon.

He discovered that once these antibodies disappeared from the blood, you could be certain the patient was developing AIDS. He published a paper with these findings in January 1986 in the *British Medical Journal*, admitting that he wasn't sure why the antibodies disappeared as a person became sicker.

Could it be that antibodies were disappearing because the B cells that make them were exhausted? Or was it because the virus was churning out so much p24 and the antibodies were sticking to it? He figured if antibodies were clumped around the protein, the test might not be able to detect them.

He answered those questions toward the end of the year and published a second article in the *British Medical Journal* in December. It's when the virus is replicating rapidly and churning out lots of p24 protein that the antibodies disappear from the blood, he said. What's more, he proved that p24 was bad news. Lots of p24 in the blood meant the virus was making a lot more copies and that the patient would soon succumb to AIDS.

With every lesson, Joep made remarkable advances in the understanding of HIV and its effect on the human body. One experiment triggered another, each answer leading to more questions.

By identifying the very particulars of the virus, its proteins, enzymes, and anatomy, Joep and scientists like him exposed its weaknesses. With these newly identified targets, he helped ignite the search for chemicals that would attack HIV at its viral Achilles' heel.

Researchers from around the world took these discoveries, and like locksmiths carving keys they studied the shape of the virus's vulnerabilities and searched for chemicals that would latch onto HIV and stop it replicating.

On the hunt for new medicines, Joep experimented with a drug called suramin, which was used to treat the parasite that causes African sleeping sickness. He injected suramin into ten patients and looked to see if it worked. It didn't. It only made his patients claw at their skin and wrap their arms around their aching bellies.

One discovery worried him more than others. He learned that HIV didn't just multiply inside white blood cells, it snuck into organs and hunkered down for months or years, far away from detection. It was exploiting a protective strategy that some organs had evolved.

The immune system can be a volatile beast. Angered by invading bugs, it wages all-out war. It floods infected wounds with immune cells and sticky antibodies. Inside the eyeballs or the brain, organs with little room to swell, this immune storm can wreak havoc. A swollen brain jammed against the hard shell of the skull can cause coma and death quicker than some infections. That's why these organs evolved ways to protect themselves from the immune system. But HIV uses this ancient strategy to turn sensitive organs like the eyes, brain, breasts, and testes into sanctuary sites, places where the virus can hide out.

Joep discovered that even when the blood seemed absent of HIV, a person might be infected with the virus. HIV wasn't flowing through their veins, it was tucked away inside lymph nodes and lurking deep inside the brain ready to wake up from a long nap.

Joep and Heleen married in the second year of his PhD at a ceremony attended by the who's who of Dutch science. Between champagne toasts and dancing, Joep and his mother-in-law played matchmaker, cajoling Peter Reiss to talk to a young woman who was friends with Heleen's family. The pair would eventually marry.

Joep and Heleen had their first child, Anna, the next summer, and their son was born in 1987. They named him Max for the Czech writer Max Brod, the author of nearly a hundred books and the best friend and biographer of Franz Kafka.

Children delighted Joep as much as the literary figures he named them after. Anna and Max were inquisitive, wide eyed, and beautiful. He wondered if he stayed long hours in the lab just to deepen the ache of missing them, to make the return home taste even sweeter.

When Max was one, Heleen gave birth to their second daughter, Maria, and they moved with the three children to a house in Muiderberg, a village outside of Amsterdam. Fatherhood deepened his drive to fight the epidemic, and Heleen gave up nursing to raise the children while he split his time between the ward, the lab, and home. His mind was filled with case control studies and lullabies.

One day when he was riding the tram to work, he was engrossed in his thoughts and nearly missed his stop. Hopping off near the AMC he watched as the tram chugged away and realized he had left something on the seat next to him. His PhD thesis.

Another time he left the thesis in a briefcase on the doorstep of his mother-in-law's house. The poor woman traipsed around the neighborhood in search of the papers eventually finding them in an alleyway.

His thesis was a compilation of eight of the most important papers he had published in the mid-1980s—and he had plenty to choose from. In just four years Joep published nearly two dozen articles in some of the most prestigious medical journals in the world, and he landed significant discoveries in the fields of virology, immunology, and clinical care. His productivity was fueled by his own ambition and the collective need to learn more about AIDS.

Most students reformatted their published articles for their PhD thesis so that the final printed booklet didn't look like a compilation of the studies that appeared in medical journals. Joep's friends wondered why he didn't do the same. It wasn't the only tradition he eschewed. At the end of their PhDs, Dutch students often print a card with a dozen or so bullet points outlining their key findings. Ten of the points are serious summaries of experiments, but another three or four are absurdities thrown in to make the PhD examiners chuckle.

Karel Koch, Joep's friend and mentee on the wards, added quips about the differences in American and Dutch culture to his PhD card as well a joke about Albert Heijn, the Dutch supermarket chain. Joep was witty and should have made a card, his friends said, but he had more important work to do. They felt like they were missing out on his jokes because he didn't want to follow tradition.

On the morning of Thursday, November 5, 1987, Karel and Hans Sauerwein, the chief of medicine, drove Joep to a forest east of Utrecht. They got out of the car and walked into the woods. The plan was to distract Joep, to take his mind off the starched shirt and stiff tuxedo he would wear that afternoon when he faced a panel of stern professors. They would interrogate his work, the way he had set up his experiments and interpreted the results. It was PhD defense day, and his was the first Dutch thesis on AIDS.

A few hours and many packs of Player's Navy Cut cigarettes later, they emerged from the forest and drove back to Amsterdam. Joep changed into his tuxedo in Karel's flat, and they walked along the canal to a dark, seventeenth-century church in the center of Amsterdam.

The Oude Lutherse Kerk, or the Old Lutheran Church, was where University of Amsterdam PhD students defended their PhDs. Joep stood at a pulpit and explained his work. The event was open to the public, but the pews were mostly filled with familiar faces.

He spoke for fifteen minutes and took questions for half an hour. There was nothing he couldn't answer. He was softly spoken but confident and anticipating the party that Karel had planned. As soon as the proceedings were over, he raced to Karel's apartment and switched his black pants and jacket for casual slacks and a shirt. It was party time. He didn't notice Karel swooping up the jeans and t-shirt he had worn to the forest that morning.

Karel had arranged the party at de Industrieele Groote Club, a wood-paneled gentleman's club in Dam Square. When they arrived, Karel slipped on the clothes that Joep had discarded earlier and acted as Joep in a skit with Hans Sauerwein, Joep's supervisor. They mimicked his outbursts and sarcastic remarks and the sheepish way he offered books as gifts when he upset his friends.

Bottles of red wine were drained, and jokes were made about his excessive enthusiasm to publish his work. They chided him for losing his PhD thesis—twice—and needing his mother-in-law's help to find it. Everyone laughed, especially Joep.

The AIDS ward opened on the sixth floor of the AMC at the end of 1985. Joep and his colleagues quickly inhabited the sixth floor unit on the northwest side of the hospital, their white coats beacons against the cool green walls.

The sixteen-bed ward was divided into twelve rooms, four of them housing two beds, while eight rooms housed only one bed, giving patients the utmost peace and privacy.

Sven Danner was in charge of the ward. He had been asking for a dedicated space for his patients for years, but the hospital's managers had said no. They were worried about creating too many divisions within the hospital.

That wouldn't be the case, said Sven. He had already assembled a crew of neurologists, pulmonologists, dermatologists, and other experts to help him deal with the many faces of AIDS.

What the new ward lacked was a head nurse. In October 1989, the hospital placed an advert in *de Volkskrant* newspaper. Jacqueline van Tongeren applied. She was unlike any nurse they had ever met. Born in Indonesia to a British mother and a Dutch father, Jacqueline was worldly, compassionate, and charming. And she was stunning. Silky brown hair framed an oval face. Designer frocks clung to her slim figure.

Her mother, Pamela, had been a radiology technician from Surrey when she met Bart, Jacqueline's father. Bart operated radios in the Dutch army and had a degree in Indonesian studies from Utrecht University, paid for the by the Dutch government, which needed Malay and Arab speakers to work in the colony. The son of a preacher, Bart would not have been able to afford an education without government subsidies.

Pamela and Bart met in Trafalgar Square on May 8, 1945, Victory in Europe Day, two people in a crowd of thousands who had gathered to celebrate Winston Churchill's announcement that the war was over.

Bart was waiting for a ship to take him to Indonesia. Pamela promised him she would write—and she did. They exchanged long letters for two years before Pamela moved to Indonesia to marry Bart in 1947. She became head of the radiology department at a local hospital, but they had to leave abruptly in December of 1949, when Indonesia won its battle for independence. Jacqueline was five months old.

They arrived in Amsterdam broke and discombobulated. And Pamela was putting on weight. "It's because of the bread we eat in Holland," Bart said. But she wasn't fat, she was pregnant. Their son Philip was born in

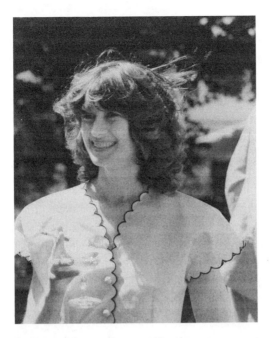

Jacqueline van Tongeren

1950. They gave him the nickname Flip after Bart's wartime code name. Sandra, their third child, was born in 1958.

Bart took up work as a printer and distributor for *Het Parool*, a resistance newspaper that was formerly illegal. To take their minds off the austere times, they took the kids to Amsterdam's art auction houses and picked out the paintings they would buy if they had the money.

Jacqueline did well in school and ballet classes but struggled with anorexia as a student at Utrecht University, where she studied Italian. She began thinking about nursing when she was married to her second husband. The couple owned an art gallery in Amsterdam called Wending. It was doing fine, but nursing seemed a better fit for her caring nature. Besides, the economy was tanking, and a gallery didn't seem like a stable source of income. Surely there would always be jobs for nurses.

Jacqueline began nursing training at the Slotervaart hospital in March of 1981, just months before the first AIDS patients would walk through the doors and onto her ward. She had a particular interest in neurology, neurosurgery, and cancer medicine and took extra classes in those subjects when they were offered. By 1987, she was head nurse of the AIDS ward. But the Slotervaart hospital was in financial trouble.

"Despite really enjoying my current job, I need a change and a new challenge," she wrote in elegant cursive in the application letter for the job at the AMC. She liked the Slotervaart hospital and had spent years refining its nursing protocols so that patients received good care and the nurses didn't burn out. But the hospital was facing budget cuts, and the AMC offered a bigger, better-resourced department.

She was the most unusual candidate for the job at the AMC. By the time she walked into the hospital for her interview with Jan and Jaap, she had worked as a translator of Italian literature, an art curator, owner of two galleries, a realtor, a restorer of historical monuments, a fine pastry chef, and of course, head of nursing at the Slotervaart hospital's AIDS ward.

"Are you sure you want to hire her?" Jaap said to Jan after Jacqueline aced her interview. "I mean, just look who she's married to."

Jacqueline was married to Adriaan Venema, a famous and controversial Dutch playwright and author who liked to pick public fights with prominent writers by making accusations about their behavior during World War II. Through essays and news articles, Adriaan made enemies of much of the Dutch literati.

Jacqueline and Adriaan owned the Wending art gallery, but Adriaan was capricious and engaged in multiple affairs. By the time Jacqueline interviewed for the job at the AMC, she and Adriaan were separated. She was dating an artist by the name of Joop.

Jacqueline had a penchant for fine art and complicated men—mercurial men, the kind of men who skipped polite conversation, dove straight into intellectual discussions, and lost their cool until she unleashed her charm and brought their tempers under control. The Dutch called them *sterk in je schoenen*, or strong in their shoes. Not macho men but resolute men with strong minds and opinions.

Before her marriage to Adriaan, Jacqueline had been married to an architect who was a controlling and unfaithful man. So it was no surprise to her friends that she was falling for the softly spoken, often shy doctor with the short temper, expressive face, and love of literature who she worked with on the AMC AIDS ward. Joep was not cantankerous like Adriaan, nor was he controlling in the way of Kees, her first husband. But he was emotional, intellectual, and enthralled with literature. And that was just the way Jacqueline liked it.

Joep and Jacqueline riffed off one another. His passion coupled with her ability to manage people and projects made them a dynamic pair on the ward. In 1990, the Dutch government gave the AMC money to set up the National AIDS Therapy Evaluation Center and the Virologic Evaluation Unit. Joep was to direct NATEC, which meant coordinating studies at twenty different Dutch hospitals, each of them designated specialist AIDS centers. Jacqueline was the glue that kept the organization together.

She liked that Joep was professional but not afraid to show his feelings. Like his father, he simply could not hide his emotions. He scuttled between patients and the lab, and Jacqueline would see him emerge from patients' rooms wiping tears from his cheeks. He was overwhelmed by their suffering.

And he was becoming increasingly difficult to manage. Frustrated at the hospital's managers, he fired off angry letters calling them stupid and complaining about the lack of funding for AIDS research. "You are blind, you can't see the importance of the work we do here," he wrote.

"Who does he think he is?" the managers would yell, descending on Sven's office, waving papers and spitting grievances. Sven would patch up the crisis until Joep sparked the next fight.

Sometimes Joep would show Sven a letter before he sent it, seeking his superior's approval, and Sven would say, "Joep, there is no way you can send this letter. Of course everything you say is right but if you send this it will be the end of our department." Joep would send the letter anyway.

In the spring of 1987, hope arrived on the AMC's AIDS ward in the shape of a capsule. It was half white, half sky-blue, with a navy band around its middle and an imprint of a black horse raising its hoof.

AZT was an anticancer drug made by Jerome Horwitz in his Michigan lab in the 1960s. Horwitz made the drug from fish sperm, and it worked great at killing cancer cells in a test tube. But when he injected it into mice with leukemia it made no difference, and he had thrown AZT onto the medicine junk pile, calling it a disappointment.

Twenty years later, researchers at the NIH were trying AZT out again, this time on the blood of AIDS patients. They got the drug from pharmaceutical company Burroughs Wellcome, who had made a batch for testing. They were calling it Compound S.

Both sets of scientists found that Horwitz's drug blocked HIV enzyme reverse transcriptase from turning HIV's RNA into DNA.

When a person swallows AZT the body turns it into a molecule that looks a lot like thymidine, one of the four bases in our DNA. AZT acts like a phony version of that base. It tricks reverse transcriptase into using it instead of actual thymidine. But when the enzyme adds AZT into a chain of DNA, the chain gets stuck. No more bases can be added, no more HIV can be made.

This was great in theory, but it had to be tested in humans. Between February and June of 1986, Dr. Margaret Fischl at the University of Miami enrolled two hundred and eighty-two HIV-positive people in a study to test AZT. The trial was almost delayed when Burroughs Wellcome ran into a manufacturing problem: it didn't have enough fish sperm to make the medicine.

The trial was based in twelve clinics across the United States. Half the patients were given AZT and the other half a sugar pill. The study was double-blind, meaning neither the patients nor the doctors knew who was getting which pill.

People in the study were given beepers that went off every four hours, reminding them to pop a pill. In concert halls and in bedrooms, during coffee breaks and in the middle of the night, the beepers sounded the alarm.

The study was meant to last six months, but four months in, nineteen people taking the placebo pill had died. One person had died in the AZT group. An independent review board looked at the early data and said it would be unethical for the study to continue with so many people dying in the placebo group. They stopped the study after four months. Only fifteen people had received the full six-month course of AZT.

The new drug was described as the light at the end of the tunnel. There were celebrations in homes, clinics, and the offices of Burroughs Wellcome. Finally, there was hope for those suffering with the devastating disease and something for doctors to prescribe.

It usually takes around a decade for a new drug to work its way through the testing process and the FDA's regulatory hoops. There are phase one, two, and three clinical trials; there are meetings about the trials. There are periods where the public is shown the data and allowed to comment and ask questions.

HIV changed that. AZT went from lab shelf to medicine cabinet in less than two years. The FDA approved the drug in March of 1987, four months before Dr. Fischl's results were published in the *New England Journal of Medicine.*

Not everyone was impressed by that study's results or convinced that AZT was a wonder drug. Seventy-five patients in the placebo group had AIDS, said critics, and all of them suffered *Pneumocystis carinii* pneumonia. Some of them died because of it. Why had they died of a treatable lung infection? some doctors and activists asked. Why were the causes of death listed in the study different to the list sent to the FDA? One person's cause of death was simply listed as "AIDS," and no autopsy was performed.

Activists and journalists used the Freedom of Information Act to uncover details of the trial. They learned that some patients thought they could tell who was given AZT and who was given placebo because of the way the pills tasted. Desperate for treatment, some patients mixed their pills with the pills of other patients in the trial in the hopes that they would all end up getting some of the real medicine.

There were notes showing that many patients in the AZT group had repeat blood transfusions because the drug had damaged their bone marrow. Dr. Joseph Sonnabend, a South African infectious disease doctor working in New York, wrote a critique of the study and sent it to the *New England Journal of Medicine* and the country's top doctors. No one responded. They were so desperate for a treatment, he said, that they had lowered the bar for scientific integrity.

Sonnabend was one of a few voices asking why patients were given such high doses of AZT. Some worried about the toxicity of the drug. But the scientists leading the study said that so-called side effects were linked to AIDS, not AZT. A later study showed the drug worked at half the dose used in the trial.

Joep had his own doubts about the trial, and he questioned the excitement over the discovery of a single drug. It wouldn't be enough to fight AIDS, he thought, and then there were the horrible side effects.

One of the problems with AZT is that while it likes to interfere with HIV's DNA, it can mess up human DNA, too. Patients taking the drug in the study suffered dizziness, fatigue, headaches, nausea, and muscle pain. The drug got into the bone marrow, the place where blood cells are made, and messed up their production so that patients felt weak from anemia. Side effects were so intense for some that they stopped taking the medicine.

Soon after AZT came two more HIV medicines. Both targeted the enzyme reverse transcriptase. Didanosine was approved in 1991 and zalcitabine in 1992. One in three people who took zalcitabine suffered damage to their nerves so that their fingers and toes tingled and went numb. One in four people taking didanosine suffered the same. The drugs could also cause ulcers in the mouth and esophagus, diarrhea, headaches, and pancreatitis.

Still, there was a widely shared feeling of jubilation. At least there were options. At least people were dying more slowly.

Joep didn't join in the celebrations. Jumping on the first thing that worked was absurd. Yes, patients were suffering, but treating HIV with only one drug would be a disaster, he said. Just look at what happened with tuberculosis. Treating TB with one medicine seemed to do the trick at first, but the bug quickly adapted to the drug and outwitted it.

It was the battle with TB that showed the benefit of combining drugs to fight a deadly infection. So why were we attacking HIV with just one medicine? Better to wait until more medicines were discovered and then give patients a potent drug cocktail.

His peers thought he was crazy.

The call came one evening. His patient Ruud was frantic on the other end of the line. Ruud's partner, Raul, had moved back to Mexico City after being diagnosed with HIV in the Netherlands. Raul wanted to be closer to his family, but his family called Ruud to say something had gone terribly wrong.

Raul's in a bad way, they said over the phone. He's aggressive, agitated, and he won't let us take him to the doctor. Ruud put down the phone and called Joep. I've got to go and get him, he said. But I'm afraid to go alone.

They flew to Mexico City the next day. Mexico was hosting the World Cup, and the Spanish football team was staying in the same hotel as Raul. Joep and Ruud navigated the crowds and the extra security checks and walked up to his room.

They found him pacing in a white wedding gown, a long, lacy train of fabric trailing behind him. He was babbling in Dutch and Spanish. Dozens of boxes of Chanel No. 5 perfume were stacked against the walls.

They tried to calm him down, but Raul was excited. He had discovered a cure for AIDS, he said. And then he dashed to the bathroom hoisting fistfuls of white satin above his waist. Besides AIDS-related dementia, he was suffering severe diarrhea.

Ruud coaxed Raul out of the wedding gown and into more comfortable clothes, but he couldn't convince him to take the medicine that Joep was transferring into a syringe.

They pretended the medicine was a vitamin solution that would give him a boost of energy. Satisfied with that suggestion, he offered his arm, and Joep injected him with the so-called vitamin solution. It was a sedative. They needed Raul to sleep so they could hatch a plan.

Joep was convinced that getting Raul to Amsterdam would save his life.

They had the best neurologists and psychiatrists there, he said to Ruud, doctors accustomed to seeing young men whose brains were addled with HIV.

But how would they get Raul to the airport? And even if they managed that, how would he handle a thirteen-hour plane ride? Raul might rouse somewhere above the Atlantic Ocean and dance along the aisles, wafting Chanel No. 5 and news of a revolutionary AIDS cure through the business-class cabin.

Ruud rested with his partner, and Joep rifled through the papers he had brought in a briefcase. He began to type a letter, a medical certificate of sorts. It said that Raul needed emergency medical care in Amsterdam and that he was medically cleared to fly.

When Raul woke, Joep sedated him with another dose of the fake vitamin solution, piled him in a taxi, and they drove to the airport.

The security official looked up from the letter, eyed the trio and looked down again. He folded the letter and waved them through the checkpoint. Joep and Ruud sandwiched Raul in the middle seat between them. His head was lolling, his mouth gaping. At four-hour intervals Joep injected him with a sedative.

But they were spotted: the flash of the hypodermic needle, the glint of the foil cap. Passengers began to crane their necks. They watched the sleepy, sickly looking man who was being propped up between a strange pair who kept prodding him. Someone complained to the air steward. "They are trying to kill him!" one man shrieked.

No, Joep explained to the angry crowd on the plane. He was trying to save his patient's lover's life.

There was another man in Mexico who needed his help. Han Nefkens was a reporter for the Dutch radio station, VARA, and a stringer for America's National Public Radio when he was diagnosed with HIV in 1987.

It happened through a homeopath. Han was coughing, and his chest felt tight. He put it down to the Mexico City smog and went to see a homeopath. He was a Dutch man wearing brown sandals, and he insisted that Han get a bunch of blood tests, including one for HIV.

"Why?" said Han. "Is it because I'm gay?"

The homeopath insisted it was a precaution.

"Fine," said Han. "I'll do it because you insist, but I'm telling you now it's going to be negative."

He refused to believe the results until a second test came back positive.

Doctors in Mexico City told Han there was nothing they could do to help. AZT had been approved by the FDA, but it wasn't available in Mexico so Han flew to the Montrose Clinic in Houston, where doctors checked the number of T cells in his blood, a way of measuring the immune system's strength.

He had four hundred and forty T cells in each cubic milliliter of blood, less than the five hundred or more they would like to see, but not a bad result. They started him on AZT, a huge step, since it was confirmation and a daily reminder of his status. And the list of side effects unsettled him. So far, he felt fatigue but nothing else. What if the AZT made him ill?

He took the pill, but when he went back to Houston three months later his T cell count had dropped to three hundred and thirty. Doctors told him about a clinical trial at the NIH, where patients were being treated with an experimental treatment called interferon.

Han wasn't sure. He spoke to a friend, who suggested he speak to a Dutch doctor. Han flew to Amsterdam to meet Joep.

"Don't join the clinical trial," Joep said at their first meeting in April 1988.

Han was taken aback by the doctor's bluntness.

"It's a noble thing to volunteer in a trial but interferon will make you feel sicker, and it won't work against the virus."

Joep didn't offer platitudes or promises, only truths, including how little was known about experimental treatments. Han was disarmed by Joep's honesty, his willingness to admit the unknowns. It was the beginning of a lifelong friendship.

More than a decade later, when Han lay in Barcelona, his brain swollen, his eyes rolling back in his head, Joep flew from Amsterdam to rescue him. He arrived at the hospital and hauled Han to the airport, where they boarded a flight to Amsterdam the same day. It was at that point that Han felt he might escape death. He was in good hands now, the hands of a man who would fight for his life.

Joep had been right. Treating HIV with one medicine turned out to be a disaster. Monotherapy did buy some AIDS patients a few extra months, maybe a year, but within eighteen months the virus grew resistant to the medicines.

In the presence of one drug attacking just one part of the virus, HIV could learn its enemy. It evolved to survive. Every time the virus replicated and made copies of itself, it made particles that were each slightly different from one another. The particles that could best fight the medicine were the ones selected to replicate. It was survival of the fittest, and only the strong survived.

Joep's lab mate, Dr. Charles Boucher, was studying exactly how the virus became resistant to the medicines. He looked at the blood of eighteen people in Roel's cohort. All of them had been taking AZT, although a few had to lower the dose because the medicine was toxic.

Charles discovered that the gene coding for reverse transcriptase, the enzyme that AZT blocked, was mutating. The virus was making changes at four specific spots in the enzyme, and that's how it was protecting itself from AZT.

Charles took blood from the men every four months and noticed that sometimes the virus mutated to a type that could survive AZT and then it would revert to its original state. And then he watched as it mutated again. HIV was constantly shifting, as if it was figuring out which disguise was most elusive.

Charles discovered that resistance developed more quickly in people who were sicker compared to people who took AZT before they had severe symptoms.

He found that at any one time the men's blood was populated by millions of virus particles, each with its own mutations. AZT and the virus were battling inside the body, and the virus was mutating to become resistant.

On the ward, tension was growing between Sven and Joep. The two men respected each other enormously, but their egos clashed at every meeting. They talked about it over a coffee one day, admitting that it was difficult to work together. I feel like it's impossible to give you the space and freedom that you need, Sven told his protégé.

Joep felt the hospital was closing in around him. His fourth child, Martha, had just been born, and his ambitions were growing bigger. He began traveling around Europe and to the United States to meet with physician-scientists who, like him, were at the cutting edge of this new epidemic.

His frustrations were obvious to everyone who worked with him, so it wasn't a complete surprise when he announced he was leaving the AMC, but where he was headed came as a shock.

Students and doctors huddled in the stairwells and around microscopes.

"Have you heard? I couldn't believe it!"

"He won't last long at that place. Not with his temper," they whispered.

Sven heard the news and felt relief. He needed space from Joep and knew that his mentee had been searching for other opportunities. But even he was shocked about his destination.

He had overheard phone calls from Dutch universities trying to lure him away from Amsterdam. Joep had turned them down. There were even rumors of offers from drug companies who wanted to hire Joep as a full-time medical advisor. He had turned those down, too.

Joep was leaving his family and the Netherlands for a place that nobody would have guessed. They wondered if he would ever return to Amsterdam.

5 *Unusual Bureaucrat*

Coffins lined the roads leading into the city. Barefooted men and women hawked the caskets out of rusty trucks and zinc-roofed shacks. Mahogany-brown coffins stood next to pale brown ones, neat crucifixes carved into their lids. Flimsy cardboard coffins were cheapest but notorious for bringing funerals to a sudden stop when the thin base crumpled and a body fell out. Some of the sturdy wooden caskets were only two or three feet long, unvarnished, unmarked.

A white car trundled past the coffin sellers, past goats chewing at the side of the road and children riding bicycles in flip flops. Joep was staring out the car window, his eyes bouncing over the lush green vegetation, the red earth and the children shrieking. It was August, rainy season was on its way, and the air above Kampala was heavy with expectation.

His new job at the World Health Organization didn't officially begin until September, but there was no time to wait. His soon-to-be boss called and sent him to Uganda in August of 1992. A crisis was brewing in East Africa.

The WHO had botched its initial response to AIDS by not responding at all. Leaders there didn't officially acknowledge AIDS until 1983. That year an internal WHO memo mentioned the epidemic but said there was no need to participate in the global AIDS response. The disease "is being well taken care of by some of the richest countries in the world where there is the manpower and the know-how and where most of the patients are to be found," the memo said.

Two years later, when the virus had spread to every region of the world, the director-general of the WHO, Dr. Halfdan Mahler, told the scientific and medical community not to worry about the growing epidemic. He suggested they keep HIV in perspective to other health concerns.

The next year, he said he had made a mistake. "I definitely admit to a gross underestimate," he told reporters. "Everything is getting worse and worse in AIDS and all of us have been underestimating it, and I in particular...I thought wait and see, maybe it is not as hot as some are making it appear."

By the time Joep switched his lab in Amsterdam for an office in Geneva, fourteen million people were infected with HIV, almost a million people had died of AIDS, and the virus was still creeping up and up toward its peak.

AIDS was now the leading cause of death for men in their midtwenties to midforties in America, where a million people were HIV-positive. Cities like Miami, Chicago, and Austin were dimming their skylines in remembrance of the dead. Half a million people were infected in Europe, three million across Asia, another million and a half in Latin America and the Caribbean.

But it was in Africa, below the sandy belt of the Sahara, that the virus got its deepest foothold. Only 10 percent of the world's population lived in sub-Saharan Africa but nine million people there were infected with HIV. Poverty, racism, and the aftermath of colonialism and war fueled the epidemic's expansion across countries like South Africa, where a person was dying of AIDS every minute.

The trip to Uganda was Joep's first journey into Africa, his first time seeing the way HIV destroyed things beyond skin cells and lung tissue. Here, it wiped out communities, ripped apart families, and devalued currencies.

His driver navigated the road from Entebbe airport to the city, passing the botanical garden and the pebble beaches that lined Lake Victoria.

HIV was creeping along its shores, where women with hungry children and empty pockets sold their bodies to fishermen in exchange for tilapia. The virus was hitching rides in the blood of truck drivers and making pit stops at dusty motels along Uganda's trucking routes.

One in three Ugandans was suffering with "slim disease," the local name given to AIDS because of the way it stripped flesh from the bones. Most of them were mothers and fathers. They died in their twenties and thirties and left behind a nation of orphans and bewildered grandparents.

Where there is dying and desperation, there are humans who feed on despair. Scavengers who jostle among the mourners looking for ways to exploit their grief, to make a quick buck and line their own pockets. For every epidemic, there is a charlatan peddling a magical elixir. Some of them sit on curbs trading tinctures for coins, others wear shiny suits and sell prayers. But the most dangerous of all snake oil salesmen are the ones who masquerade as scientists and politicians. They hide their greed behind white coats and official titles.

In 1990, a Kenyan scientist said he had discovered a miracle treatment for AIDS. Dr. Davy Koech was director of the Kenya Medical Research Institute, known as KEMRI. Davy fed hundreds of AIDS patients a wafer dipped in medicine he called Kemron. It was a wonder drug, he said with a wide smile.

Patients who chewed on the wafer put on weight and grew stronger, Davy said. According to him, their symptoms disappeared and some even tested negative for HIV after ten weeks of treatment. He published one set of findings in the *East African Medical Journal* and a second article in an American, peer-reviewed journal, the *Journal of Molecular Biotherapy*. In that paper he said eight patients treated with Kemron for just six weeks cleared HIV from their blood.

News spread quickly, and people flocked to Kenya from around the world. They emptied their purses for Kemron. "There are some people who would do anything to get it," a young Kenyan woman told reporters. "They would sell their houses, go to any extreme."

Outside a Nairobi clinic, a thirty-two-year-old man waved cash and a prescription for Kemron. A doctor in Nairobi said he could get Kemron for free. He told a reporter, "Now today they are saying 100 shillings for every tablet. The amount I have is 400 shillings, enough for four days."

Within weeks of Davy's announcement, a bootleg version of Kemron was for sale in Uganda and Kenya. Fraudsters were scamming off the scammers.

But Kemron wasn't new, and it wasn't discovered by Davy. It was another name for interferon-alpha, a chemical the body makes when fighting an infection. It was already known that high doses of interferon-alpha injected into cats could treat feline leukemia, and a chewable version of the drug was synthesized in Texas in the 1970s by Joseph Cummins, a white veterinarian. Joseph had developed the drug to treat respiratory infections in cows. In fact, it was Joseph who supplied the drug to Davy. The pair had met in 1989, when Cummins traveled to Kenya to study cattle. He likely told Davy during that trip how he fed his mother-in-law mucus from a cow's nose when she was diagnosed with malignant melanoma and how the mucus, which in his experiments seemed to contain interferon, had cured her.

Interferon-alpha wasn't new in the world of HIV. It was approved for the treatment of Kaposi's sarcoma in the United States in the 1980s. High doses of the drug had to be injected under the skin for the lesions to disappear. Davy was claiming that swallowing small amounts could clear HIV.

American scientists had considered the same idea as Davy a few years earlier, and a group at the NIH had begun testing interferon-alpha as a potential treatment for HIV. When AZT was approved, they started a trial comparing AZT with interferon-alpha, but their experiments were only halfway through by the time Davy announced his spectacular results.

The scientists read his studies, paying close attention to the methods sections. They noticed how Davy didn't test Kemron alongside AZT to see how it compared to a drug known to fight HIV. He didn't include a placebo group, either. His results couldn't be trusted.

Davy stood by his claims and was backed by the Kenyan government. He said he was the first person to feed wafers laced with small amounts of interferon-alpha to AIDS patients and he would patent his discovery. When Joseph Cummins, the Texas veterinarian, heard this news he threatened to sue.

Kemron was more than a medicine. It was an emblem of Kenyan nationalism, a symbol of African scientific achievement. Despite no decent evidence to show that it worked, it was celebrated as a triumphant discovery made by scientists in the nation plagued by AIDS. Any hint of skepticism about Kemron from the West was seen as a racist attempt to suppress Black success.

In America, where AIDS was the number one killer of Black men and women, the Nation of Islam heralded Kemron as a cure for HIV. AZT was a poison, it said in the pages of its newspaper, the *Final Call*. Editorials accused the WHO of purposefully spreading HIV in Africa and censoring African scientists who had discovered a cure. The Nation of Islam alluded to a "conspiracy of silence" about Kemron in the white media.

"The racist white press" was "cabalistically [ignoring] this amazing discovery," said editors of the *New York Amsterdam News*, one of America's oldest Black papers. Kemron was being overlooked because white people believed that Black scientists "could not possibly have come up with an effective therapy or cure for AIDS that has eluded white scientists and researchers," they said.

Dr. Abdul Alim Muhammad, a physician and former spokesman for the Nation of Islam leader Louis Farrakhan, received a federal grant of more than two hundred thousand dollars to treat patients with low-dose interferon-alpha at his Washington, DC, clinic. He sent a supply of the drug to NWA rapper Eazy-E when he was diagnosed with AIDS in 1995. Interferon-alpha arrived at the star's Los Angeles hospital, where friends said he perked up after taking the treatment. He died of AIDS a few weeks later.

With news of an apparent wonder drug, there was pressure on the WHO to test interferon-alpha and say something, anything, about its efficacy. Senator Ted Kennedy even sent a letter to one WHO official urging him to hurry up and do a study. In October 1990, a few months after the Kenyan president publicly proclaimed the effectiveness of Kemron, Davy flew to Geneva. After he met with experts at the WHO, they released a statement saying that interferon-alpha was still experimental and still not proven to work against HIV. The WHO would conduct its own trials, they said.

The Kenyan government was not pleased. President Daniel Arap Moi announced that Kemron had cured dozens of AIDS patients and saved them from imminent death. The vice president said a local factory would begin to manufacture the drug so that the miracle treatment would be widely available. HIV patients, desperate and destitute, continued to sell their belongings and empty their pockets for Kemron.

Ending the Kemron crisis was Joep's first WHO assignment. Officials at the agency wanted to test the drug in six hundred patients in three countries: Zimbabwe, Zambia, and Uganda. But there were problems recruiting patients in Zimbabwe and Zambia, so they asked a physician in Uganda, Dr. Elly Katabira, if he could find six hundred patients in his Kampala hospital. Sure, said Elly. Finding AIDS patients was not a problem.

Joep's journey from the airport to Elly's hospital took just over an hour. Mulago Hospital sat at the top of a hill south of Makerere University, where Elly was a lecturer. It was the largest hospital in the country, with close to nine hundred beds. On April 10, 1987, when thousands of Ugandans were infected with HIV, Elly took a room in the hospital's polio ward and turned it into an AIDS clinic. He had returned to Uganda from England in 1985 right as his country's AIDS epidemic was exploding. He had become Uganda's leading HIV doctor and researcher.

Elly walked out of the white brick hospital as Joep's car climbed up the hill, creeping toward the six-story building surrounded by a cluster of older clinics. The car door opened and two lanky legs emerged. Joep stood up, straightened his crumpled shirt, and smoothed his hair. He introduced Elly to his coworker Jos Perriens, who was also from the WHO.

Elly stood a few inches shorter than Joep. He was a stocky man with a square jaw and a gap-toothed smile. He shook Joep's and Jos's hands and led them onto the ward.

It smelled of bleach and rot. The hot stagnant air stuck to their skin like a shroud. There was no air conditioning. Metal bed frames creaked beneath the weight of groaning bodies, two or three people crammed onto mattresses designed for one. Cadaverous men and women whimpered on the floor in between the beds, some of them cradling babies on their bony chests. Patients were crying out in pain and calling for help, but there was not enough staff to help them. A select few had family members who served as carers. They emptied bedpans and cradled their loved ones' weary heads, staring into their glassy eyes as they fed them sips of water.

There was no clean water on the ward, no gloves or pillows. Patients brought their own sheets and blankets from home, if they could afford them. Joep fought back tears. He had never seen an AIDS ward with as many women and children as men.

He followed Elly through the ward to the outpatient clinic, where a woman waited with a baby strapped to her back. She hitched up her dress to show them a deep wound between her vagina and anus. An ulcer was eating away at her flesh, its flat white center outlined by an angry red rim. It was herpes. AIDS was wrecking her immune system and as her defenses grew weaker, the ulcer grew bigger.

Joep had seen plenty of AIDS patients with herpes in the Netherlands but none with an ulcer as large or as deep as this one. He waited for Elly to give the woman pain medicines and acyclovir, a drug that treats herpes. Elly had neither. The woman walked out of the clinic empty-handed and Joep sat in silence. He was stunned by the pain and injustice of what he had witnessed. He couldn't hold back tears any longer.

His mission in Uganda was to check on the interferon-alpha study. Elly's team had recruited five hundred and fifty-nine patients, who had been randomly assigned to one of two groups: people in the first group were given low-dose oral interferon-alpha, and people in the second group were given a sugar pill. The study was double-blind.

Joep checked on the trial's progress, peering at blood and serum samples to make sure they were stored properly. He thumbed through case reports, looking to see that documentation was thorough and clear. Elly had everything under control.

Sifting through the charts with Elly, he confided in him that he wasn't prepared for the suffering he witnessed on the wards. He had seen the statistics but hadn't been able to imagine human suffering of this depth, on this scale. Elly nodded.

It would be months before they had enough data to say anything meaningful about Kemron, but both Elly and Joep believed Davy's claims were too good to be true. Joep said Kemron was an expensive fake, and he cursed the doctors who sold it to dying AIDS patients.

That visit to Kampala and the beginning of his friendship with Elly was a turning point in his life, not just in his career. He was already committed to fighting the epidemic, but now he swore to never shut up about the suffering of AIDS patients in Africa. The injustice and inequality was mind-boggling. Three HIV medicines were approved by the time he visited Uganda—AZT, didanosine, and zalcitabine. None of them were on the shelves at Mulago Hospital.

He felt disillusioned with the way medicine was practiced in the West. As corpses were carried out of Mulago Hospital on stretchers, he thought about his patients back in Amsterdam, the way they complained about fatigue, diarrhea, and the inconvenience of swallowing AZT capsules every few hours.

He vowed never to tolerate the whining of Western AIDS patients again. "After seeing all of this I was unable to take care of people who complained about having to take too many pills," he wrote. He would care for patients again a few years later, but he had to be selective about who could join his roster. "I literally told several of them to find another doctor."

Sixty weeks later, the results were in. Joep and Elly announced the findings of their interferon-alpha study at the 1994 International Conference on AIDS in Berlin. The drug was useless. "In both treatment groups there was relentless progression of HIV disease," Elly and Joep said. One hundred and eight people died in the interferon-alpha group and eighty-three people died in the placebo group.

Their study was proof that Kemron was no better for AIDS patients than a sugar pill. Joep hoped the findings would put the conspiracy theories to rest. But the Nation of Islam was still countering that Kemron worked and that the US government was trying to shut it down.

Joep spoke directly to the racial element of the Kemron crisis. "This study was done in Africa by African investigators," he told reporters. "That takes away the argument that the criticism of low-dose alpha interferon is all white racism. This study was done on black people by black doctors."

But activists in the United States told Elly his study wasn't trustworthy, precisely because it was done by Africans in Africa. Elly flew to New York to testify in front of a panel of experts. Joep was too furious to speak. He was afraid he would explode during his presentation and told Elly he should give the talk alone. Elly could control his temper.

Four more studies by the WHO showed similar results. The Kemron crisis was finally ending. With his first site visit a success, Joep flew back to Geneva to officially begin his job as chief of clinical research and drug development at the WHO. His department was housed within the Global Programme on AIDS, which had been set up in 1986 after the WHO confessed to not taking the epidemic as seriously as it should have.

Dr. Halfdan Mahler, the director-general who had said initially that AIDS was not a concern, had recruited a young, bright doctor to head the GPA. In 1986, Dr. Jonathan Mann left his job at an AIDS organization in Zaire and moved to Geneva.

Jonathan was a former Epidemic Intelligence Service officer at the CDC and state epidemiologist for New Mexico. He was adored by many public health practitioners, who admired his human rights stance and his work ethic. In just a few years, Jonathan transformed Project SIDA in Kinshasa into one of the top HIV research organizations in the world.

He was just as dynamic at the WHO, a trait that was not always appreciated at the world's largest health bureaucracy. Jonathan took the Global Programme on AIDS from a new initiative and turned it into the largest single-disease program at the WHO. Within two years the GPA raised close to ninety million dollars, more than any other WHO division. The money didn't come from the WHO's central budget; Jonathan raised it directly from donor countries. Under his leadership, the GPA began providing financial support to more than a hundred nations.

His success made some WHO bureaucrats bitter. They didn't like the press he received or the way he worked. Jonathan believed in the power of local groups and nongovernmental organizations, and he often bypassed the WHO's regional offices and got straight to work setting up national AIDS programs in developing countries.

He framed HIV as a social justice issue, not just a medical one. In countries like the United States, national polls showed that the majority of the public supported the idea that people with HIV should be locked up in quarantine camps. Politicians in some countries spoke about tattooing everyone who tested positive. Jonathan's supporters said his work at the WHO was directly responsible for putting those kinds of ideas to rest.

Complaints about his media savvy and work style had landed on Halfdan's desk from the beginning of the GPA, but Halfdan had left Jonathan to get on with his work. The trouble started in 1988, when Halfdan left and a new director-general was appointed.

Dr. Hiroshi Nakajima was a seasoned bureaucrat who had worked at the WHO for more than a decade. He was not a fan of Jonathan's celebrity status. Hiroshi began to interfere with the GPA's budget and even messed with Jonathan's travel plans.

Jonathan quit in 1988. His resignation sent ripples around the AIDS world. Just seven years into the epidemic with so much work ahead of them, many felt they were losing a leader who cared passionately about the rights of people living with AIDS, a person who was fighting tirelessly for change at the highest levels.

Jonathan was replaced by Michael Merson, an American doctor and former Epidemic Intelligence Service officer. Michael hired Joep as well as Peter Piot, a Belgian AIDS doctor. Peter would be his assistant director and Joep's day-to-day supervisor.

Peter had met Joep once before when he visited Amsterdam in the 1980s to meet the Dutch quartet. He admired their work and had good memories of Joep.

In Geneva, they became fast friends. Both men hated authority and laughed at their new shiny offices inside the world's biggest health bureaucracy. Both spoke Dutch as their mother tongue and adored the writing of Belgian poet and novelist Willem Elsschot. Both were desperate to escape their hometowns as boys. Peter was born in Keerbergen, a small Belgian town about an hour's drive east of Nieuwenhagen, the village where Joep was born.

They talked about books and red wine, infectious diseases and women. Peter thought Joep was a *bourgondier*, a connoisseur of the finer things in life. Literature and language was their bond, but they spent long hours talking about their marriages. Both were going through rough spots.

They shared frustration at the injustice of the epidemic and the ineptitude of governments. Why did you join the WHO? Joep asked Peter, and Peter described how his AIDS patients in Antwerp, many of them Congolese, died by the dozens. He was tired of not being able to save them. Joep nodded.

They never fancied themselves as bureaucrats—Peter lasted three months in the Epidemic Intelligence Service before he fled to academia, unable to tolerate the red tape at the CDC—but they hoped that inside the belly of the planet's health agency they could effect real change. Both men were desperate to save the world.

Saving the world requires paperwork. Joep struggled to keep up with the copious amounts of forms and files he was supposed to fill in after every trip. He forgot to file travel expenses, misplaced his mandatory travel forms, and would march over to Peter's office to complain that he wasn't getting reimbursed on time.

He broke the rules constantly. He wrote directly to drug companies, asking them to fund clinical trials in the developing world, a tactic that landed Peter in trouble with his seniors.

"You can't just go to drug companies like that," Peter said.

"Why not?" said Joep. "It doesn't matter if the cat is black or white as long as it catches mice."

He sent angry memos on official WHO letterhead to prestigious professors and institutions. "Dear Sir," he wrote to one AIDS conference organizer. "I am writing to thank you very much for your invitation to this important meeting. I am not looking forward to the presentation from Dr. A as I've heard him give the same talk before. I will be bringing a box of rotten tomatoes to Dr. B's talk so I can throw them at him while he speaks. Yours sincerely, Joep Lange."

He sent a copy of the memo to his friend Sean Emery in Sydney. Sean wrote back congratulating Joep on the elegance of his prose. He added: "This is why your career at the WHO will not last."

But it did. For three years Joep commuted on his bicycle from an apartment in Prévessin, a small French town a thirty-minute ride from Geneva, to the WHO headquarters on Avenue Appia. He took flights from Geneva to Kinshasa and Johannesburg, to Rio de Janeiro and Washington, DC. He went back and forth to the Netherlands to visit Heleen and the children. Martha was only a baby, but he would take Anna and Max back to Geneva for short trips, where they played in his office while he worked.

Heleen opted to keep the kids in Muiderberg to avoid disrupting their schooling and play life, which she nurtured with playdates and trips to the IJsselmeer, Holland's biggest lake, where the children learned to swim and sail. She preferred to focus on the quotidian of raising children and kept her distance from Joep's professional life, with its constant travel and dinner engagements. He would have to look elsewhere to share his professional achievements.

But mostly, he was haunted by the trip to Elly's hospital. Images of babies strapped to the chests of dying women were hard to shake, and he didn't want to forget. He told his steering committee at the WHO that their main focus should be preventing HIV in children and keeping their mothers healthy. Half a million children were becoming infected with HIV every year, most of them picking up the virus from their mothers as they entered the world. Passage through the vagina during delivery was the riskiest time.

One of the first clinical trials he proposed in his new role was to test a drug in pregnant women with HIV. The drug was still in the experimental phase, so it had the name BI-RG-587. It worked by attacking reverse transcriptase, the enzyme that turns HIV's RNA into DNA, allowing the virus's genes to slip into ours. Unlike AZT, which parades as a phony piece of DNA, BI-RG-587 attacks reverse transcriptase from a different angle. It sticks to the enzyme's weak spot and knocks it out.

A few months after he settled into his new office, Joep flew to Washington to visit the drug's maker, Boehringer Ingelheim. The company was meeting with a network of experts called the AIDS Clinical Trials Group, or the ACTG. It sponsored most of the major studies on HIV and promising treatments.

The medicine and the company were familiar to Joep. He was already working with Boehringer Ingelheim to test its drug on patients in Amsterdam as part of the company's international trials.

Now he was desperate to try the drug in the developing world to see if it stopped HIV spreading from pregnant women to their babies. Joep told the group it was unethical to experiment on poor people before testing the drug to make sure it was safe and didn't harm the fetus. He suggested those safety studies should be done in the developed world, places like the United States, where high-tech equipment can monitor the health of the baby and where help is at hand if pregnancy complications arise.

The company was interested, but it had different priorities. First, it wanted to finish testing the drug on adults and fill out the reams of paperwork needed to get into the FDA's approval process. Joep's prevention trial would have to wait.

On his trips to sub-Saharan Africa he saw that AIDS patients in different places were vulnerable to different diseases. In Amsterdam, he'd gotten used to hearing the dry, raspy cough of patients with *Pneumocystis carinii* pneumonia. But in parts of Africa, fewer than 4 percent of AIDS patients developed that disease.

There were other peculiarities, too. People with AIDS in West Africa were more likely to die with a chest full of tuberculosis and a brain riddled with toxoplasmosis compared to patients in Europe or even in East Africa. In Côte d'Ivoire, half of the AIDS patients who had an autopsy had TB inside their bodies.

It turned out that so-called slim disease was really a deadly combination of AIDS and TB. HIV left the body wide open to infection with the bacteria that causes TB, and it bloomed inside the lungs, brains, kidneys, and spines of people with AIDS. TB was the leading cause of death on the AIDS wards in places like Mulago Hospital.

Treating TB became his next mission. Using the standard TB treatment combination of four drugs, the first letter of each medicine spelling out the word RIPE, he started trials in people with HIV. When those were successful, Joep showed that a medicine called isoniazid, the "I" in RIPE, could prevent AIDS patients from getting sick with TB.

One summer, Joep and his colleague Jos, flew from Geneva to Bangkok to check on some study sites. On a whim, they decided to pay a visit to a young doctor in Chiang Mai, a city in northern Thailand. It was here that Thailand's epidemic raged hardest. Chiang Mai was just south of the Golden Triangle, one of Asia's biggest opium-producing regions. More than one hundred thousand Thai were HIV-positive, many of them drug addicts in the north who became HIV-positive by sharing needles.

That afternoon, Joep and Jos turned up at a cinderblock office in Chiang Mai with no invitation and no announcement. They walked into the three-story building and said they wanted to see Dr. Chris Beyrer.

"Dr. Chris, two *farangs* are here to see you," said the secretary using the Thai word for foreigners. "They don't have an appointment."

Chris was glad for the company. He was thirty-four years old, fresh out of an infectious disease residency at Johns Hopkins University in Baltimore, and he had been sent to Chiang Mai as field director of Hopkins's Preparation for AIDS Vaccine Evaluations Center. At the time, it was thought a vaccine was a year or two away from discovery.

Chris led the WHO officials, who didn't quite look or behave like WHO officials, into his windowless office. There were white tiles on the walls, a drain in the center of the floor, and a faint stench of dead animals that hung over their heads. His office was a former animal research lab and the site of many bloody massacres of monkeys and guinea pigs. Local staff refused to work there alone in fear of meeting *pii*, spirits that possess the human soul.

Chris had been in Thailand just over a year and was fluent in Thai because many of his colleagues did not speak English. He was happy to have a conversation in his mother tongue, especially with two men a few years his senior who said they had heard good things about his work.

Joep was laid back and instantly likeable, not stuffy like a WHO bureaucrat, and before he knew it, Chris found himself sharing sad memories. He talked about Luther, the man he had fallen in love with in medical school who had tested positive for HIV when Chris was in his final year.

Luther died in 1991 after a long illness. In the months after his death, Chris lost half a dozen friends to AIDS. He was devastated, didn't know what to do with his grief, and retreated from social life, locking himself up in a house on Fire Island.

HIV was a job to some people. They treated HIV patients because it paid the bills. They searched for the virus through a microscope when they were really looking for endowed professorships and tenure. So many people were jumping on the HIV bandwagon, planning on making a career out of the epidemic, and Chris could smell their ambition a mile away.

Joep was not one of them. It was obvious he cared from their first conversation in the windowless room and their long chat on the rooftop, where they smoked Camel Lights. It was obvious that he cared from his reaction during their visit to Chiang Mai University Hospital, where they walked through wards full of emaciated men and women, their skin covered in black and red sores the size of dimes.

The stinging, visible stigmata of AIDS in Thailand was penicilliosis, infection with the fungus *Penicillium marneffei*. The disease was so rare that only fifty or so cases had ever been reported in the world, and here they were surrounded by more than a hundred patients with the illness.

The fungus wasn't only erupting on their skin. It was spreading through their veins causing a fungal sepsis and making their livers and spleens balloon. The treatment was awful. Patients had to spend weeks in hospital hooked up to an IV that pumped amphotericin B into their blood. The antifungal liquid was toxic, could damage their kidneys, and worse still, the fungus came back time and time again after it had been treated.

Joep wondered if oral antifungal medicines would work. If they did, it would allow patients to treat themselves at home without the painful infusions they received in hospital. Soon after that meeting with Chris, Joep set up a collaboration with Dr. Thira Sirisanthana, director of the Research Institute for Health Sciences at Chiang Mai University. They compared the effectiveness of three types of medications, each of them taken by mouth.

Their study was a game changer. They discovered that oral itraconazole cured the infection. The best part was that patients could keep taking the medicine at home to prevent the fungus from ever returning.

The real game changer would have been HIV medicines, drugs like AZT and didanosine, which were only available to white and wealthy AIDS patients in countries like England and the Netherlands, not in places like Chiang Mai or Kampala. In those places, they were playing a waiting game, trying to buy time as they fought off one bug after another.

It wasn't the first opportunistic infection that killed you, it wasn't even the second. But by the time the third illness hammered your worn-down body, there was nothing left to fight with.

When he was back in Geneva, a letter arrived from Amsterdam. It was from Sven. His mentor had been wracked with guilt when Joep left, but the initial relief was chased by a nagging feeling that he had lost his right-hand man. "I'm sorry," Sven wrote. "I'm begging you to please come back. I was short-sighted." Sven had figured out a strategy that would allow them to work together without pushing each other's buttons and getting in each other's way. "I'll focus on the patients and studies in Netherlands and you can focus on the rest of the world," he wrote. "Please come back."

Joep smiled. He was touched by the honesty and tenderness of those words. He held on to the letter until 1994, when things began to fall apart at the WHO. It seemed the Global Programme on AIDS would not survive another year. Fierce clashes between senior staff were destroying it from the inside out. One report said, "Interagency rivalries and the behavior of some WHO staff undoubtedly provided ammunition to those supporting the demise of GPA."

Donors began to have doubts. Countries that had made large donations to the program said they wanted to set up their own programs. Joep and Peter's boss, Michael Merson, couldn't stand to work with Hiroshi Nakajima any longer. The same director-general who had left Jonathan Mann with no option but to quit was driving Michael out, too. He left Geneva in 1994 and became a professor at Yale.

As the GPA crumbled, a new bureaucracy was born. UNAIDS, or the Joint United Nations Program on AIDS, was inaugurated in 1996, and Peter was appointed executive director.

He didn't try to recruit Joep to UNAIDS. He knew that Joep was tired of the red tape and inertia. There seemed to be no drive to get HIV drugs to the people who needed them most. Joep decided he would leave the WHO in 1995. As he packed up his office, he challenged Peter on his decision to stay.

"What are you doing here? You've become too polite and too political," he said.

"Don't fight with me," said Peter. "We're on the same side, aren't we? I am not the enemy."

6 *Trials*

Once upon a time a heretical priest and a pair of young lovers were trapped in an authoritarian state. Baltasar, a wounded soldier was besotted with Blimunda, a peasant girl with mystical powers. The priest was an aviation pioneer. He built a flying machine, a bizarre contraption of metal plates, ropes, and cranes, to escape the Spanish Inquisition. But as the trio planned their liberation, Blimunda hesitated. Eyeing the rig, she asked the priest: How will the Passarola fly? The priest had studied in Holland, where he learned of a novel energy source. Human conviction will act as fuel, he told Blimunda. How can freedom be won without it?

Joep put down the novel and sipped his Heineken. These days he found himself drawn to José Saramago's fantastical tales. The Portuguese author was a breaker of rules, a defender of love, and he knew a thing or two about plagues and the powerless. In his books, society dissolved when diseases spread and thousands suffered under the rule of gods and monarchs who cared little about the poor. José knew about being an outsider, too. The writer was fired from his job as a journalist and exiled from Portugal, accused of being a blasphemer, a communist, and an anarchist.

Joep wondered if he had exiled himself. He left the World Health Organization on the cusp of a breakthrough. Two new classes of HIV drugs were about to be approved, meaning HIV could now be ambushed from three different angles. Finally, there was a chance that science could conquer the virus.

He had been saying it for years, since 1988 in fact: HIV was a wily foe, and it should be treated the same way tuberculosis had been managed since the 1950s—with a cocktail of potent medicines, not just one.

So it was interesting to see in 1996, the year after Joep left the WHO, Dr. David Ho's bespectacled face gracing the cover of *Time* magazine. The American AIDS researcher was celebrated as the magazine's Man of the Year for his "championing" of combination therapy.

But Joep had bigger problems than being overlooked for a magazine award. Many scientists hadn't listened to Joep when he suggested they wait for combination therapy. They had jumped on AZT. Patients from Amsterdam to Anacostia were fed the pills alone or in combination with drugs that attacked HIV the same way as AZT. That strategy turned out to be a disaster. Not only was it useless, it was dangerous.

When patients were given AZT on its own or with one other pill, they perked up for a while, maybe for a few months, maybe even a year, and then they fell sick again. The drugs stopped working. In the presence of a few, weak drugs, HIV fought back with a vengeance and grew stronger.

Worse still, a person infected with a strain of HIV that was resistant to AZT could find the entire class of reverse transcriptase inhibitor drugs was useless. They might even be resistant to medicines they had never taken.

A few months after Joep quit his job at the WHO, a new drug was approved and with it, a whole new class of HIV medicine. Saquinavir gave hope to people whose infection was resistant to AZT. It was licensed on December 6, 1995, less than fourteen weeks after the drug's maker, Hoff-mann–La Roche, submitted the application to the FDA.

Saquinavir was the first drug to attack HIV from a completely different angle. It didn't block reverse transcriptase, it crippled another of the virus's enzymes—protease. When HIV is deep inside a human T helper cell and the cell is churning out the proteins HIV needs to make more virus particles, protease snips the protein strands into the right shapes and sizes. Without protease, HIV's proteins clump into useless sticky balls. Some virus particles are made, but they are not infectious.

Next came nevirapine—the eighth anti-HIV drug and a third class of medicine. Nevirapine blocked the same enzyme as AZT but in a different way. It didn't pretend to be a building block of DNA. Instead, it stuck to reverse transcriptase at one of its weak spots and left the enzyme flailing. Nevirapine was better than the other HIV medicines at penetrating the brain and spinal cord, where HIV would sneak in, replicate, and leave people feeling nervous, confused, and forgetful.

Nevirapine was new on the market but familiar to Joep. It was the drug made by Boehringer Ingelheim Pharmaceuticals and formerly known as BI-RG-587, the pill he had wanted to test at the WHO to see if it protected babies from being born with HIV. He had already helped the drug company test the medicine on Dutch patients, and now that there were three classes of HIV drugs, he was designing a trial to play around with different combinations of the new and old medicines.

Joep wanted to prove that he had been right about combination therapy all along. He partnered with friends and colleagues in Australia, Canada, and Italy, doctors like Mark Wainberg, David Cooper, Julio Montaner, and Stefano Vella, as well as colleagues in Amsterdam including Peter Reiss, to compare different drug combinations and see what worked best.

Across the four countries, Joep's team divided over a hundred patients into three groups. One group received AZT and nevirapine, another group got AZT and didanosine, and the third group received all three drugs.

The patients taking three drugs saw the biggest improvements. Their white cells recovered, the virus withered. Triple therapy—treatment with all three classes of drugs—was the clear winner. The study, which was given the nickname INCAS, was a turning point in HIV treatment and a personal win for Joep. He could say, "I told you so," to all the naysayers, the doctors who had been using mono and dual therapy when he had been telling them to wait.

He was like the heretical priest on the Passarola looking down as the airship lurched and jerked and eventually lifted into the night sky. Conviction was his fuel.

But the celebrations were short-lived. As quickly as fresh drugs arrived, so did bad news. Dr. Doug Richman at the University of California,

San Diego had given nevirapine to twenty-four patients and a combination of nevirapine and AZT to fourteen others. Within seven days, patients in the nevirapine monotherapy group developed resistance to the drug. Even patients in the dual therapy group became resistant, although it took them a few more weeks.

The problem was how quickly HIV evolved. Every second, dozens of new virus particles were made, giving the virus ample opportunity to tinker with its genes. It was crafty, selecting for virus particles that had mutations that protected them from the medicines, no matter that the medicines were brand new and had taken millions of dollars to develop.

Joep, Peter Reiss, Charles Boucher, and others did their own experiments in Amsterdam. They gave nevirapine to twenty patients and watched as they perked up and their HIV levels plummeted, but the amount of virus in their blood soon shot right back up to where it had been at the beginning of the experiment. Old drugs, new drugs—they stopped working.

When Charles peered at HIV to see how it was disguising itself, he found tiny mutations in its reverse transcriptase enzyme. HIV was making the smallest of changes, switching one amino acid for another, and that was enough to render the medicines useless.

There was another problem. Nevirapine caused a rash so red and scary-looking that doctors were forced to stop some of their patients from taking the medicine. Saquinavir had nasty side effects, too. It made the heart thump to a strange beat and it clogged the arteries with fat.

They had hoped that newer drugs would be more potent and have fewer side effects, and while protease inhibitors like saquinavir and its cousin indinavir did pack a bigger punch, they did strange things to the body.

Fat bulged in bizarre places and shriveled away in others. Patients patted their potbellies and nicknamed them protease paunches or Crix belly after Crixivan, the brand name for indinavir. You could tell who was on a protease inhibitor, they said, because they looked like Big Bird, all skinny legs and bloated bellies.

At the same time, protease inhibitors made fat vanish from the cheeks and buttocks. A flat bum made it hard to sit for a long time, especially on the hard seat of a bicycle or on the bus during the commute to work. And then there were the buffalo humps that sat at the nape of their necks, solid mounds of fat that grew and grew.

Potbellies, gaunt cheeks, skinny legs, and buffalo humps. Indinavir even turned eyes yellow. These were the stigmata of HIV in the 1990s, except they were caused by modern medicines, not the virus. Bodies became billboards screaming to the world that you were HIV-positive. It felt like the 1980s, when you could tell who had AIDS by how skinny they were. Now you could tell who had HIV by looking into their eyes. Cheeks and necks and bellies told you exactly which pills they were taking.

But at least these patients have pills, Joep muttered, walking through the AMC's AIDS ward. He was back in Amsterdam after his three-year stint in Geneva. Sven, who had written to him when he was at the World Health Organization and begged him to come back to Amsterdam, was pleased his friend was home. He had even convinced managers at the AMC to appoint Joep professor of medicine. The same administrators who had been on the receiving end of the young doctor's rude memos in the early 1990s grudgingly agreed to give him the position.

He looked the part of an erudite professor, his black hair was starting to turn silver, his brow was often furrowed as he walked the hospital's corridors taking long purposeful strides. The tails of his pin-striped blazer flapped around his waist, piles of patient charts and medical journals were tucked between the crook of his elbow and his chest.

Besides, it was hard to deny his achievements. He had been chief of an entire division at the WHO and was leading some of the most pioneering HIV studies in the world. He brought prestige—and perhaps more importantly, money—to the AMC.

He also brought complaints. Those who knew him well understood that the outbursts and snarky memos were borne out of frustration at the injustice of the epidemic, but his patients didn't always understand. They were on the receiving end of some less-than-compassionate remarks. "So what you have to take so many pills? At least you have pills," Joep said to one woman who sat in stunned silence. She asked to be switched to a different doctor. Sven bowed his head, apologized, and quietly made the arrangements.

Jacqueline rolled her eyes. She had held down the fort, quietly building the AIDS ward into a center of clinical excellence while Joep was away saving the world. And here he was, back on her turf, disturbing the peace. They were opposites in that way. She left a trail of gentle smiles and peace behind her as she glided down the ward. Patients' eyes lit up, and they sat up in their beds as she approached, hoping she was coming to talk to them. She would perch on the edge of their bed, take their hands between her small, soft palms and ask, "How are you feeling today?" And then, stripping off her latex gloves to place the back of her hand on their forehead she would say, "Let's try and get you better."

She spoke to them about ballet, theater, and fine cuisine, reminding them of the foods they had enjoyed before HIV medicines stripped the lining from their guts and reduced their diets to cartons of warm milkshakes designed for geriatric patients.

Jacqueline was a glimmer of their old lives, of fancy restaurants, couture, and the latest cocktails. Even when an eye infection forced her to switch from contact lenses to glasses, she shopped for a fancy pair of cat-eye spectacles. A glint of purple flashed from the underside of the frames every time she tilted her head to laugh.

At home, she cared for her partner Joop, an older man who was sick with a lung disease that made him weak and cantankerous. She nursed him in the evenings after she clocked off from her shift on the AIDS ward, only missing him on those nights when she swapped shifts with nurses who had children. Jacqueline was quick to offer respite to her colleagues when they needed to be with their kids. She wanted children but didn't have any of her own. She would slip to the maternity ward during her breaks and listen to the gurgles of newborns, their breaths condensing in puffs of white fog against plastic incubators. She was in her midforties and wondered if she would ever be a mother. A struggle with anorexia as a teenager made it difficult to get pregnant as an adult. Her patients were her charge; she poured her energy into comforting them, listening to them talk about death and love and the toxic taste of their pills.

She told Joep how hard it was for their patients to swallow the medicines, and it wasn't that Joep dismissed the side effects of the new drug cocktails; he took them seriously, even writing about them in journals, but after seeing patients die from a lack of medicines in Uganda, he couldn't stand to hear patients complain about problems caused by pills.

In a Dutch medical journal he wrote about the hardships of three of his patients, a gay man and two straight women, all of them on drugs like saquinavir and indinavir. The padding on their buttocks and cheeks disappeared and their tummies ballooned. Their arteries were choked with fat, making them vulnerable to heart attacks and strokes. Joep described their pill problems in the case report. But at least they had pills.

"I don't want to hear about your fatigue," he said to Han Nefkens, the man who had moved from Mexico City to Barcelona just so he could be closer to Joep. Han was doing well on a regimen he mostly tolerated, but his biggest problem was a thick curtain of fatigue that clouded his brain like cheesecloth.

"Tiredness is nothing to complain about," Joep said, pursing his lips. Han shrugged it off. They were friends, and he had heard about the visits to Thailand and Uganda, about the corpses of AIDS patients carried out on stretchers, the children who died on hospital floors next to their weeping mothers.

But fatigue and fistfuls of pills were valid concerns. Toxic, complicated drug regimens were the enemy of patients and the friend of HIV. They helped the virus become resistant to the medicines designed to fight it.

The latest regimens involved chugging dozens of tablets—some as big as quarters—two, three, or four times a day. Forgetting to take a pill or taking it at the wrong time or taking it with a low-fat meal instead of a high-fat meal or mixing it with water instead of a creamy milkshake could mean victory for the virus. If the right amount of medicine wasn't constantly circulating in the blood, the virus had a drug-free window, an opportunity to wake up and rapidly replicate. It was at those times that it mutated and built up resistance to the pills.

Those bitter, bulky pills. "Is this tablet for a human or a horse?" patients asked Jacqueline, prodding the thick white discs in their hands.

They were like blocks of chalk that got stuck in their throats. Some had to be crushed and jammed into gelatin capsules. Some came as sticky syrups that made the tongue tingle and coated the back of the throat with a lining that tasted like metal. No amount of water could shift the taste.

You heaved, you spat, you drank water, you swallowed more tablets, you drank more water. And on days when you were running from the gym to the grocery store, picking up flowers and a bottle of wine for a date, feeling refreshed and on top of the world, it was the pills that reminded you, every few hours, that you weren't fine, you were infected with a virus.

Some days it was easier to take the batteries out of the pager, slide them into a drawer, push away the pills that had been emptied into Advil bottles so that no one would know what they were really for, and pretend that there were no medicines and there was no HIV.

Until there was a cure, until the virus was purged from their bodies, Joep believed combination therapy was the only way to keep people alive. He was convinced that it was key to stopping the epidemic. Every year, top HIV scientists said they were two years away from a vaccine, every year they said they were inching closer. But it was 1996, and there was still no vaccine.

They needed to work with what they had, and Joep knew that if he could simplify the combinations, cut down the number of pills, and lessen the side effects it would make life easier for patients and more difficult for the virus.

One way of paring down the combinations and making them less toxic was by switching protease inhibitors for a different class of drug. But protease inhibitors were the most potent HIV medicines in their arsenal, so he needed to be sure replacing them wouldn't give the virus reprieve. Joep designed two huge and pivotal studies to find out if protease-sparing regimens were a good idea.

In one experiment, called the Atlantic study, he gave some patients nevirapine and others the protease inhibitor indinavir. Patients who took nevirapine did just as well as those who took indinavir, even if they had begun the trial with thousands of HIV particles floating in their blood.

Another study that showed it was okay to leave protease inhibitors out of the drug cocktail was the 2NN study, which Joep designed. In that study, he compared nevirapine to a newer drug in its class called efavirenz. Both drugs blocked reverse transcriptase. There were four groups of patients in the 2NN study. Some took nevirapine either once or twice a day, some took efavirenz, and some took a combination. All patients were taking two other drugs from the same class as AZT.

It turned out that efavirenz was the slightly better drug, although nevirapine was a solid option. Combining the two wasn't a good idea. It made for a more toxic cocktail with no added anti-HIV effect. Two patients in the study died because of nevirapine. One person died because the medicine made the liver swell. Another person developed a fatal skin rash called Stevens-Johnson syndrome, a disease triggered by certain drugs. The skin blistered and peeled off in chunks until death occurred.

The two studies showed that combining nevirapine and other drugs in its class with medicines like AZT was a good option. It meant fewer pills, fewer dietary restrictions, no protease paunches or buffalo humps, less fatty buildup in the blood vessels, and fewer stomach problems. And it meant you could save protease inhibitors for when you were desperate, for when the virus had built up resistance to the other classes of drugs and you needed to call for backup.

The name given to this potent cocktail of pills was HAART, short for highly active antiretroviral therapy. HAART was born in 1996, the same year as Joep and Heleen's fifth child. He named her Ottla, after the nickname of Ottilie Kafka, Franz Kafka's favorite—and youngest—sister.

With Ottla cooing and crying at home as her mother and four siblings fussed over her, Joep's mind was focused more than ever on saving babies in the developing world. Every minute, a child was infected with HIV, most of them right as they were being born. In parts of sub-Saharan Africa, up to half of all children born to HIV-positive mothers picked up the virus as they passed through the birth canal.

Soon after Ottla was born, Joep got to work on a trial nicknamed Petra. It was designed to investigate if medicines could prevent a mother passing HIV to her baby. In South Africa, Tanzania, and Uganda, Joep's team screened more than twenty-three thousand pregnant women and enrolled nearly two thousand of them who were HIV-positive in the study. Some of the women were patients at his friend Elly Katabira's clinic at Mulago Hospital in Kampala.

The pregnant women were split into three groups. The first group swallowed AZT and lamivudine every day as soon as they reached the thirty-sixth week of pregnancy. They took the medicine during delivery and for one week after while also feeding their babies AZT or lamivudine syrup for a week.

Women in the second group took the medicines during delivery and with their babies for a week after birth, but they weren't given the medicines during pregnancy. In the third group, women were only given the medicines during delivery. They didn't receive the medicine after birth, and neither did their children.

It was babies in that third group who fared worst. They did no better than babies whose mothers didn't receive any medicine at all. But babies in the first group, born to mothers who took the drugs at the end of pregnancy, during delivery, and for a week after, were a lot less likely to be infected with HIV. Joep calculated a 63 percent reduction in babies being born with HIV in the first group. The reduction was around 40 percent for babies in the second group.

He was overjoyed. Healthy babies were being born to mothers with HIV. Each negative HIV result brought relief and conviction that the virus could be conquered, at least in some children.

But the good news did not last long. Joep and his team had been checking in on the children, meeting with them and their parents every few months. Things seemed fine at first. The babies were happy and healthy, teething and crawling. But by the time they turned eighteen months old they weren't testing negative for HIV anymore. All of them had become HIV-positive.

What had gone wrong? Had the drugs worked for a while and then failed? They had tested the children every few weeks, and those tests had been negative, so surely the drugs had worked?

The problem was breastmilk. The virus was passing through the mothers' nipples into the suckling mouths of babies feeding on their mothers' milk. It was a devastating discovery. What use was the trial, the weeks of toxic medicines, the inconvenience, and the expense if the children were HIV-negative as babies and HIV-positive as toddlers?

The obvious solution was to feed the children formula milk, but it was expensive, it wasn't on sale everywhere, and it could be downright dangerous for a baby to be seen with a bottle in its mouth. The mother must have that dirty virus, neighbors would sneer. Nasty woman. Why else would she not feed her baby with her breasts?

The other problem with formula milk was that the water used to mix it could kill a baby quicker than HIV. In countries like Uganda, parasites and bacteria in water caused a deathly diarrhea.

They couldn't tell women to stop breastfeeding, that wasn't an option. They had to give babies HIV medicines while they sipped on their mothers' milk. To test this idea, Joep designed a study nicknamed SIMBA. His team enrolled close to four hundred women in Rwanda and Uganda and gave them AZT and lamivudine toward the end of their pregnancy and for one week after delivery. Their babies were given either lamivudine or nevirapine as soon as they were born and for the whole time they were breastfed. The mothers had to carry on feeding their babies the medicine for a month after they stopped breastfeeding.

The study showed this simple drug combination could let babies receive all the benefits of breastmilk without becoming infected with HIV. With the help of the drug cocktail, the chance of the virus spreading from a mother's milk to her baby dropped from 15 percent to 1 percent.

Joep and his colleagues had to be careful how they communicated their findings. Breast is best, Joep repeated to the mothers and the clinical trial staff, even when a woman has HIV. The most dangerous scenario was mixed feeding, when babies were fed a combination of breast milk, formula, and food. Bugs in the food damaged the delicate lining of the baby's gut and made it easier for HIV to pass from the mother's milk into the baby's bloodstream.

It was a tricky intersection of science and culture, stigma and survival. Joep struggled to keep his frustration in check, but his optimism soared. Especially now that he was part of a growing global community of physician-scientists, nurses, activists, sociologists, and anthropologists who looked at HIV through the lens of social justice and human rights.

It was a global network led by people like him and Jonathan Mann, the American doctor who had been the first director of the Global Programme on AIDS at the WHO. After he quit the WHO in 1990, a few years before Joep would join, Jonathan started HealthRight International, an organization connecting health to human rights. Then he became dean of the Allegheny University School of Public Health.

Like Joep, Jonathan was pushing for universal access to health care, and at times it felt like they were making progress, baby steps of progress, but it was progress all the same. And then came the worst news Joep could imagine.

On the evening of September 2, 1998, Jonathan and his wife, Dr. Mary Lou Clements-Mann, an HIV vaccine scientist at Johns Hopkins University, boarded a plane at New York's John F. Kennedy Airport. They were headed to Geneva to talk about strategies to end the HIV/AIDS epidemic. The meetings were at the WHO and the United Nations, and their flight, Swissair flight 111, was jokingly referred to as the UN shuttle because it so often ferried UN officials across the Atlantic Ocean.

An hour and fifteen minutes after Jonathan and Mary Lou's plane took off in New York City, it crashed into the Atlantic Ocean off the coast of Nova Scotia. All two hundred and twenty-nine people on board were killed. An electrical spark from the in-flight entertainment system had ignited a fire.

The AIDS community reeled. Joep was stunned that a tragedy could suddenly rob them of two scientists leading the battle against the virus, two people in love and fighting to tell the world that AIDS was not just a medical problem, it was a human rights catastrophe. He reacted the only way he knew. He vowed to work harder.

The heretical priest in José Saramago's novel didn't build his flying contraption overnight. It had taken him many years to craft the Passarola. In secret, for fear of being burned at the stake, he hammered away, collecting information and materials. Piece by piece, with help from Baltasar and especially from Blimunda, who had the ability to capture human will, the jaunty airship had grown and with it, the trio's faith that it would save them. But that airship, powered by faith, would crash, leaving the priest bereft and the two lovers fighting for their survival.

Joep understood that life was littered with moments of joy and terror, that progress came with setbacks, and that fighting injustice took time and perseverance. Relative to other diseases, the world of HIV medicine was rapidly advancing. When Joep left the WHO in 1995, five years after Jonathan had quit, there were half a dozen drugs to fight a virus, all of which had been discovered and approved in the span of eight years. Now there were another eight drugs discovered between 1995 and the time of Jonathan's death in 1998. There were tests and treatment guidelines. It was progress built on hard work, but it wasn't enough.

The heretical priest fleeing the Inquisition had worked hard, in secret, but his story was about more than conviction. His story was about taking your ideas, the grand and seemingly impossible ones, and not letting the beliefs of others determine your fate.

Joep would have to be a pioneer. He would have to be outspoken and brave. If he wanted to extend Jonathan and Mary Lou's legacy and make sure the poorest women and children in the world had access to the best medicines in the world—a pledge he had made when he had sat with Elly in Mulago Hospital—then he would have to innovate.

He had already begun. A few months after he left the WHO, Joep was on a mountainous island in the Andaman Sea. Phuket was covered in a thick blanket of rainforest, warm turquoise waters lapped at its shores. He was sweating beneath the heat of the Thai winter that afternoon with two friends, Dr. David Cooper and Dr. Praphan Phanuphak, when the trio hatched a plan.

They had been invited to Phuket by officials at the pharmaceutical company Glaxo Wellcome. Like its competitors, Glaxo Wellcome often held medical meetings at luxury resorts like this one. Perhaps it hoped the combination of sun and fruity cocktails would blur the lines between business and pleasure.

David was an Australian immunologist who had diagnosed the first case of AIDS in Australia. Praphan was a Thai doctor who had diagnosed the first three cases of AIDS in Thailand. He was director of the Thai Red Cross AIDS Research Centre in Bangkok and personal physician to the Thai royal family. He was also in charge of escorting Hollywood royalty like Elizabeth Taylor when they visited Thailand's AIDS wards.

Both had served on Joep's steering committee at the WHO. It was there, during meetings that dragged on for days, that they became friends and shared their frustrations. Why were decisions about how to fight the epidemic in Asia and Africa made by white doctors who sat around oval conference tables in places like Geneva?

The high-tech labs where drugs were developed, the state-of-the-art clinical units where drugs were tested, and the erudite researchers given control over the clinical trials were in the places where Joep and David worked, not in Asia, which was quickly catching up to sub-Saharan Africa to become an HIV hot spot.

Close to a million Thai were HIV-positive by the mid-1990s. Many of them were injecting drug users who were mysteriously vanishing. Their dismembered bodies turned up in alleyways and on beaches. They were being murdered as punishment for their addiction.

Thailand's epidemic was worst in the north of the country in cities like Chiang Mai, where Joep had visited Dr. Chris Beyrer, a few years back. Their trip to a local AIDS ward had sparked an idea in Joep to start a trial. He had helped find which medicine was the best treatment for penicilliosis, a fungal infection afflicting half the country's AIDS patients. He wanted to do more studies like that one, studies in the places where people suffered most.

But drug companies liked their research affiliates to be in places they could easily navigate, where they understood the language and where infrastructure was familiar. They wanted drug approval agencies like the US Food and Drug Administration to have vetted the labs and staff. That was easier in Europe, North America, and Australia, they pleaded.

What the world needs is a clinical research center in Thailand, Joep, Praphan, and David agreed over beers at the Phuket resort. One that would rival the labs in London and New York. Why couldn't an emerging nation have a state-of-the-art clinical research facility?

They wanted to put Bangkok on the clinical trials map. Joep believed every person with HIV should be enrolled in a clinical trial. It was the only way to get access to the latest drugs. If they set up a clinical research center in Bangkok, Thai people could be tested, treated, and enrolled into trials, and the balance of power could be tweaked, ever so slightly.

They needed three things: money, drugs, and equipment. Who better to ask than the officials who had invited them to Phuket? Glaxo Wellcome wanted to pick their brains, but Joep, Praphan, and David were about to switch the game.

Late one afternoon, after a long set of presentations, the trio made their request. They hoped the tropical sun would warm Glaxo Wellcome staff to their request.

Perhaps it was the spicy green curry they ate for lunch, perhaps it was the promise of an evening swim in the sea. It may have been the trio's combination of aggressive persuasion (Joep), gentle charm (Praphan), and persistence (David), but Glaxo Wellcome staff said yes, they would help them set up a clinical research facility in Bangkok.

With one pharmaceutical company under their belt, it was easier to go to Glaxo Wellcome's competitors, companies like Hoffmann–La Roche and Boehringer Ingelheim, and say, "Why aren't you supporting research and development in the developing world?"

Four months after that winter meeting, Praphan was presiding over their new organization. They named it HIV-NAT, the last three letters representing the Netherlands, Australia, and Thailand. It was a humble beginning for a center that would become part of the clinical trials network and an internationally recognized facility for testing new drugs.

Praphan operated HIV-NAT out of one room in the Thai Red Cross Society's offices. Space didn't stop him and his small team from recruiting dozens of patients to a clinical trial that would begin in the winter of 1996. It would be HIV-NAT's first of many contributions to the world of HIV and AIDS.

One of HIV-NAT's early trials compared two different drug combinations, neither of them containing protease inhibitors. Besides the side effects that distressed HIV patients in the West and had Joep searching for less toxic regimens for his own patients, Thai patients couldn't afford protease inhibitors. Saquinavir cost six thousand dollars a year.

Praphan and his team recruited patients at King Chulalongkorn Memorial Hospital and Siriraj Hospital in Bangkok. They treated them with different drug combinations and checked to see how they were doing. After nearly a year of treatment, the two groups had a test to see how much HIV was in their blood.

Praphan expected to find small amounts of HIV flowing in the veins of patients on triple therapy, proof that HIV was subdued by the cocktail. But he couldn't find any HIV. He switched to a new, ultrasensitive machine, one that could detect as few as fifty HIV virus particles in one milliliter of blood. It worked. It picked up the tiny traces of HIV in their samples. He scribbled "undetectable" next to those patients' identification numbers in their lab notebooks. The medicines were suppressing HIV to the point that there was barely any virus left in the blood. Undetectable became the new goal.

Pediatric medicine often lags behind adult medicine, even as babies are held up as the most precious and fragile creatures on earth. It was the same with HIV. Doctors around the world were playing a guessing game with the doses of HIV drugs for their tiniest patients. Drug companies rushed through trials in adults so they could get their drugs approved. That left pediatricians with calculators and pencils in hand once the drug was available, working out how much medicine to give a toddler based on the dosage for a seventy-kilogram adult.

The HIV-NAT team did an experiment testing different drug combinations in the smallest humans. Praphan enrolled babies at the King Chulalongkorn Memorial Hospital who were born to mothers with HIV. He gave all the newborns stavudine and didanosine and split them into three groups, each receiving a different amount of the protease inhibitor nelfinavir.

And that was how they discovered the perfect dose of each drug. The news ricocheted from HIV-NAT's one-room office in Bangkok to clinics in Atlanta, Birmingham, and beyond.

The organization's impact was felt locally, too, and that was important to Joep and to Jacqueline. She was helping Joep manage his responsibilities to HIV-NAT while working with staff to develop nursing protocols, something she had done at the beginning of her career as a nurse in Amsterdam. She liked to work out ways that nursing staff could provide the best, most compassionate care to their patients while maintaining their spirits and not working to the point of exhaustion. Alongside Joep, she found herself taking HIV-NAT nurses and trainees under her wing. And as they recruited local staff and built their team, Joep wanted to nurture the talents of young Thai doctors and help accelerate their careers.

"Have you ever thought about doing a PhD and becoming a professor?" Joep said to Jintanat Ananworanich, a Thai doctor at HIV-NAT who had trained as a pediatrician in the United States. Jintanat had followed a residency at the University of Chicago with two fellowships at Baylor College of Medicine in Houston, even squeezing in a stint in the lab of Dr. Anthony Fauci at the National Institutes of Health. She badly wanted to do a PhD at Baylor, it had been her plan all along, but then her mother fell ill with breast cancer and Jintanat moved back to Thailand to take care of her.

"Yes," she said to Joep. "Yes, I definitely want to do a PhD."

Joep made it seem that anything was possible, but it was Jacqueline who made things happen. She was the glue that turned his ideas into diplomas. While Joep made grand plans and copious promises, Jacqueline responded to Jin's anxious emails about deadlines and vivas and paperwork. When Joep sponsored Praphan's daughter, Nittaya, it was Jacqueline who made sure Nittaya's documents were in order so that Nittaya would get her PhD.

Jacqueline had worked in one of the administrative offices at the University of Amsterdam and always knew exactly who to contact for any particular inquiry. As Joep recruited PhD student after PhD student in Thailand, Jacqueline saw to it that each of them was happy, taken care of, and on track to graduate.

Joep had an idea to let the flow of students work both ways. He suggested that Dutch students visit HIV-NAT to do research projects and learn from Praphan's team. He began the initiative with his usual enthusiasm, and soon young researchers arrived in Bangkok from Amsterdam eager to get started. Except Joep hadn't made the proper arrangements, and the Thai team was left scrambling. They pulled together money and helped pay for the students' lab work and housing.

Soon after HIV-NAT was launched, it began a yearly symposium in Bangkok to bring together Thai doctors and global experts on AIDS. Jacqueline kept the January meetings running smoothly. Praphan's phone would sometimes ring the day before the symposium and it would be Joep, explaining how he wouldn't be able to make it. "I triple-booked myself! Sorry! See you another time!" Praphan would switch the order of the speakers and find someone to fill in for his friend.

Jacqueline would follow up with calls and emails apologizing on Joep's behalf, saying that he was needed in two other places and that they should hold his head accountable, not his heart.

Their partnership was a lot like Baltasar and Blimunda's, two people committed to a cause, both passionately devoted to ending the suffering of people with AIDS—Joep with his bold ideas and tenacity and Jacqueline with her kindness and charm, which she employed to bring people on board and transform Joep's vision into a brilliant reality.

She had the capacity to tap into people's core, understand their motivations, and bring them on board. And when their peers slowed them down or said that Joep's ideas were outlandish, she soothed his temper and refocused his energy on their projects. She wanted to protect him from those who didn't understand his anger was borne of frustration at the injustice of the epidemic, at the lack of ingenuity and faith coming from his fellow physician-scientists. They should be innovating, he said, not maintaining the status quo.

When the Passarola crashed, Baltasar and Blimunda wandered together in search of refuge and Baltasar wondered: perhaps some deeper and more mysterious sacrament sustains this union. They wondered that, too: how their bond would withstand the forces of suffering and ambition.

One day, Baltasar returned to the airship, and as he was fixing it, the Passarola took flight unexpectedly, with him hanging off a wing. Blimunda went in search of her love, scouring Portugal for nine long years until she found Baltasar at an auto-da-fe, a public ritual where heretics were tortured during the Inquisition. Baltasar was bound to a stake, about to be burned, and Blimunda could not save him. All she could do was capture her darling's faith.

7 *Denial*

The president of South Africa was in denial. He wondered, maybe HIV didn't cause AIDS?

It was the spring of a new millennium, six years after the end of apartheid, and his people were dying. South Africa had the biggest and fastest-growing HIV epidemic on the planet. Two thousand South Africans were becoming infected with the virus each day, thousands were dying of AIDS every week. Yet their president was not convinced that HIV was the cause.

He called for a meeting. Three dozen of the world's preeminent scientists gathered in a conference room in the capital, Pretoria, on May 6, 2000, half of them believers, the other half denialists. Question 1a on their agenda: "What causes the immune deficiency that leads to death from AIDS?"

The discovery of HIV, a scientific certainty that had been settled in 1984, was up for debate. The president kicked off the meeting that morning with a poem. "Since the wise men have not spoken, I speak that am only a fool," he said, reading the first line of Patrick Henry Pearse's poem, "The Fool." The room of international scientists shifted nervously in their seats.

There was Bob Gallo, the American virologist who had helped discover HIV seventeen years earlier. A few seats from him was Peter Duesberg, a German scientist at the University of California at Berkeley, who said HIV was harmless and didn't cause AIDS. There was David Rasnick, an

American biologist, who believed AIDS didn't exist and would disappear if you just stopped testing for it.

Luc Montagnier, the French virologist who had feuded with Bob over the discovery of the virus now in question, was sitting at the table. Near him was Dr. Elly Katabira, Joep's friend from Uganda. Elly was sitting up straight in a dark gray suit listening to the president of South Africa recite Irish poetry.

> *Yea, more than the wise men their books or their counting houses or*
> *their quiet homes,*
> *Or their fame in men's mouths;*
> *A fool that in all his days hath never done a prudent thing.*

Dr. Helene Gayle was listening, too. Helene was a pediatrician and public health expert from the US Centers for Disease Control and Prevention. Sitting across the table from her was Dr. Salim Abdool Karim, head of AIDS research at the South African Medical Research Council and Dr. Joseph Sonnabend, the South African doctor working in New York who had raised questions about the early AZT trials.

They had all seen the five-page letter that the president of South Africa had sent to Bill Clinton, Tony Blair, and other world leaders the previous month, defending his right to question what science had proven— that HIV destroyed the immune system and caused AIDS. In that letter, the president pointed to major differences between the HIV epidemics in America and Africa and pushed back on the imposition of Western ideas on an African nation.

"As Africans, we have to deal with this uniquely African catastrophe," he wrote in the letter, which was leaked to the *Washington Post*. "It is obvious that whatever lessons we have to and may draw from the West about the grave issue of HIV/AIDS, a simple superimposition of Western experience onto African reality would be absurd and illogical."

He was rejecting a one-size-fits-all approach to a disease that looked different in his part of the world. In Europe and America, HIV was mainly—but not exclusively—spread through sex between men, whereas in Africa, heterosexual sex was the driver of the epidemic. Africans with AIDS died quicker and in larger numbers than AIDS patients in the West, and they suffered with different opportunistic infections; tuberculosis was rife.

Years later, he would say he hadn't been in denial and was simply exercising his right to question a commonly held belief. His detractors were conducting a carefully orchestrated campaign of condemnation, he wrote in the letter, where he reminded the world leaders that until recently his nation had been under the brutal rule of a white minority that violently suppressed Black leadership and thought.

"Not long ago, in our own country, people were killed, tortured, imprisoned and prohibited from being quoted in private and in public because the established authority believed that their views were dangerous and discredited. We are now being asked to do precisely the same thing that the racist apartheid tyranny we opposed did, because, it is said, there exists a scientific view that is supported by the majority, against which dissent is prohibited."

He defended his right to engage those discredited and dangerous scientists, people like Peter Duesberg and David Rasnick, who had been mocked by many of their peers, including Joep. Joep hated them, and he didn't mince his words. This is ludicrous, he had said, reading Peter's and David's papers. These men are stupid.

But the president of South Africa wanted to hear them out. "In an earlier period in human history, these would be heretics that would be burnt at the stake!" he wrote in the April letter. "The scientists we are supposed to put into scientific quarantine include Nobel Prize Winners, Members of Academies of Science and Emeritus Professors of various disciplines of medicine!"

He was right. Peter Duesberg was one of the first scientists in the world to describe the physical features of retroviruses, to decipher their genes and show that they transformed healthy cells into cancer cells. Without his legwork, it might have taken Bob Gallo and Luc Montagnier much longer to discover that HIV causes AIDS.

The controversy began in 1987, when Peter published a paper in the journal *Perspectives in Cancer Research*. Retroviruses don't kill cells the way HIV seems to kill T cells, he argued, therefore the cause of AIDS had yet to be discovered.

The next year he published an article in one of the most respected journals in the field, *Science*. It was titled "HIV Is Not the Cause of AIDS," and it listed six ways that Peter believed HIV broke the cardinal rules of biology.

It isn't found inside every person with AIDS; it doesn't cause AIDS if injected into chimps or accidentally into humans; it doesn't infect enough T helper cells to account for their dramatic decline in AIDS patients; and if HIV causes AIDS, then why do AIDS patients have high amounts of antibodies to HIV in their blood? Surely those antibodies would protect them from the virus causing any more damage? Peter said.

His arguments were quickly dismantled by his peers, but he remained a tenured professor at Berkeley and a member of the prestigious National Academy of Sciences. His name was even floated for the Nobel Prize, although he never won.

Sitting close to Peter in the Pretoria conference room was the minister of health, Dr. Manto Tshabalala-Msimang, a South African woman who had trained in medicine in the Soviet Union. She had earned the nickname Dr. Beetroot for her claims that AIDS was best treated with root vegetables. Beer was good, too, she said. She called AZT "toxic" and backed Virodene, a potion made with the powerful industrial solvent, dimethylformamide, which is used to make synthetic leather, among other things.

Virodene was "hopelessly unconvincing," Dr. Salim Abdool Karim had said to reporters two years before he listened to the president of his nation recite Irish poetry at a meeting in Pretoria. In the late 1990s, Manto and other ministers were pushing the solvent as a treatment for AIDS. "Like everyone else, I am baffled by the government's motivation," Salim said.

While she blocked pregnant women from using medicines to prevent HIV spreading to their babies, Manto stood behind an herbal concoction the color of strong tea called Ubhejane. It sold at roadside stalls in old plastic milk cartons beneath signs that said "HIV/AIDS clinic." Liters of the potion would disappear within hours of stall owners setting the cartons on a rickety table and declaring themselves open for business.

Secomet V was another herbal tonic enthusiastically supported by Manto. It was made from the extract of red clover and sold under the name Ithemba Lesizwe, meaning "Hope of the Nation." Meanwhile, Manto was accusing doctors of poisoning and murdering their patients with AZT.

Years later, a Zimbabwean doctor at Harvard would sift through the minister's words and the president's speeches, rifle through their policy documents and check the minutes of their meetings to tally the death toll of their actions. Pushing beetroots and herbal tonics and blocking pregnant women from taking HIV medicines cost the lives of three hundred and thirty thousand South Africans.

While the two-day meeting in Pretoria got underway, another set of deliberations was about to rock the boat. In May 2000, five drug companies met with five UN agencies, including the World Health Organization and the UN Children's Fund to form a public-private partnership. Their goal was to roll out HIV treatment programs in developing countries.

Around that table were representatives from Boehringer Ingelheim, Bristol-Myers Squibb, GlaxoSmithKline, Merck & Co., Inc., and F. Hoffmann–La Roche, some of the biggest and most powerful drug makers. They were promising to cut the cost of their HIV drugs in countries with the highest rates of HIV—countries like South Africa.

They called themselves the Accelerating Access Initiative and planned to work with governments and local organizations to put pills in the hands of the poor. So far, most drug company support in the developing world centered on HIV prevention, not treatment. Pills were considered too costly and complicated for poor people.

Both sets of meetings were in anticipation of the AIDS event of the year. On July 9, twelve thousand people slipped conference badges over their heads and filed into Durban's International Convention Center. It was day one of the International AIDS Conference. The theme that year was "Breaking the Silence."

Joep was pacing up and down in his hotel room. He was president-elect of the International AIDS Society, the twelve-year-old group that ran the biennial conferences. There had been calls to boycott this gathering because it was in Durban and activists, doctors, and scientists the world over were outraged at the South African president's and health minister's treatment of people living with HIV. But the IAS committee had pushed on, and Joep was glad. They had been organizing these gatherings since 1985, and this was the first time in history that the conference was being held south of the equator.

To reach the doors of the convention center, you had to walk through a lively crowd clapping their hands and singing songs in Zulu. A group of women wore white t-shirts emblazoned with "HIV-positive." A man waved a green placard with white writing that read, "Pharmaceutical companies, stop making profits at the expense of people's lives." Inside the convention center, AIDS activists passed around banners and black armbands. On blackboards they had painted in large pink letters: "No to silence." "No to fear."

Bodies crammed into overcooled ballrooms and smaller breakout sessions. There were dozens of presentations happening at the same time, but the word on everyone's lips was "access." Finally, Joep's peers were catching up to what he and AIDS activists had been saying for years—that every HIV-positive person should have access to lifesaving medicines.

Scientists from Bangladesh and Tanzania pinned posters onto boards in one of the exhibition halls. Graduate students balanced laptop computers on their knees in the corridors and rehearsed their talks. There was excitement about new drugs and new medical strategies and even a promising vaccine.

And then President Thabo Mbeki walked onto the main stage. "You are in Africa for the first time in the history of the International AIDS Conferences," he said smiling. It was the opening ceremony in a cricket stadium two blocks from the convention center. Moments earlier, fireworks had erupted in the night sky. The smell of sulfur hung above the heads of a few thousand conference attendees, who sat on white folding chairs watching the president speak. A live telecast broadcast the ceremony to people watching inside the convention center and around the world.

The president's voice boomed through the loudspeakers: "It seemed to me that we could not blame everything on a single virus." People in the audience began to shake their heads, some shouted: "No! No! This has nothing to do with our lives!" "Shame on you!"

He was rejecting white domination, celebrating independence, and sharing his vision of an African renaissance. He warned them not to over-estimate the ability of an AIDS conference to bring about change and said that poverty, not a virus, was the biggest killer of his people.

"Poverty is the main reason why babies are not vaccinated, why clean water and sanitation are not provided, why curative drugs and other treatments are unavailable and why mothers die in childbirth," he said.

But this was not the message the audience wanted to hear. They had come to Durban to talk about AIDS, to learn about AIDS, to fight AIDS. They wanted to know why he wasn't making HIV drugs widely available and why his ministers were promoting herbal tonics instead of proven medicines. Hundreds stood up from their white chairs and walked off the cricket pitch.

In the weeks before the gathering, more than five thousand of the world's top doctors and scientists, including eleven Nobel laureates, signed the Durban Declaration, a two-page treaty that said HIV causes AIDS and that the controversy over this simple, proven fact could cost lives.

The Durban Declaration was a direct rebuttal to the president's and health minister's remarks and to the words of Peter Duesberg and David Rasnick. It was published in the journal *Nature* on the first day of the conference and the scientists had hoped that on this stage, in front of a global audience, the president would reverse his stance and say definitively that HIV causes AIDS and that antiviral medicines treated the infection. The president finished his speech. He did not say any of those things.

And then a tiny figure appeared on the giant platform. Big, doleful eyes scanned the crowds, the cameras, the television monitors. Nkosi Johnson gripped a microphone as big as his forearm and smiled. A red AIDS ribbon rested on the lapel of his thick blue blazer, shiny blue trousers, two inches too long for his legs, hung over green and white sneakers.

Nkosi was eleven years, five months, and six days old and the longest surviving child born with HIV in South Africa.

When Nonthlanthla Daphne gave birth to Nkosi in a township east of Johannesburg in February 1989, her baby boy was one of seventy thousand babies born with HIV that year. Nkosi was skinny and agitated, Nonthlanthla was growing weaker. She searched for help in an AIDS center in Johannesburg, where she met Gail Johnson, a white South African woman, who adopted Nkosi.

It was Mommy Gail who broke the news to Nkosi one day in 1997 that his mother had died of AIDS. Around the same time, she was trying to enroll him in a school, but teachers and parents united to block Nkosi from getting an education. Gail had disclosed Nkosi's AIDS status on the school's admission forms, and it had caused an uproar. The public fight to let Nkosi go to school thrust him into the spotlight and launched him as an international spokesperson for children living with AIDS.

Nkosi lifted the microphone to his lips and leaned his head forward. The audience waited in silence. "I just wish that the government can start giving AZT to pregnant HIV mothers to help stop the virus being passed on to their babies," he said, his left hand waving in the air on each syllable. The audience clapped and cheered and Nkosi's lips stretched and revealed a satisfied, toothy grin.

He told them how much he missed his mother, how she had loved him but could not care for him. She was poor and they were both sick. People in the audience tried to stifle their sobs out of respect for the child who was still speaking. They wiped the tears streaming down their faces.

"When I grow up I want to lecture more and more people," Nkosi said, sharing his plans of touring the country—if Mommy Gail gave him permission.

Nkosi would die eleven months later. He was twelve years old.

AIDS was a second apartheid. There were two HIV epidemics in South Africa: the kind that killed Nkosi and his mother and the kind that spread among the white elite, the lawyers and entrepreneurs, men who could write angry letters demanding powerful drugs and doctors. Men like Edwin Cameron, a justice of South Africa's High Court who delivered

the first ever Jonathan Mann Memorial Lecture at the Durban conference. It had been two years since Jonathan's death on Swissair flight 111.
The loss still stung.

Edwin was a middle-aged white man. Literate, visible, powerful. I
am here and healthy because of medicines, he said, his voice strong and
clear. He was taking medicines that most HIV-positive South Africans
could not access. Joep knew every statistic that Edwin was spelling out,
but each one felt like a blow to the head. Nine out of ten people with HIV
live in places where there is barely any treatment for their illness, Edwin
was saying, and Joep shook his head.

"This is not because the drugs are prohibitively expensive to produce,"
he said. "They are not." Edwin blamed pharmaceutical companies for their
drug-pricing structures and the international patent and trade systems
that shielded them.

It was one thing for Edwin to stand behind a podium that day, to deliver a rousing message about hope and human rights, it was another for
a Black South African woman to do the same. A few days after Christmas
in 1998, Gugu Dlamini was at her home a few miles away from where
Edwin was speaking at the International AIDS Conference. Gugu was
thirty-six years old and open about her HIV status. In fact, she had just
spoken about her life on the radio on World AIDS Day, hoping to dispel
the stigma surrounding the virus.

A few days after the radio interview, an angry mob descended on
Gugu. Her neighbors slapped and threatened her. Many people have
this thing, one man said, but they keep quiet. On December 28, a crowd
stoned Gugu to death.

There was no one to protect Gugu in her township, KwaMashu, a
township formed by the apartheid state in a province where one in three
people were now HIV-positive. "Gugu Dlamini was not silent," Edwin
told the audience. "She paid with her life."

He shared something Jonathan had said in a speech at the International AIDS Conference four years earlier. "He said that of all the walls
dividing people in the AIDS epidemic, 'the gap between the rich and the
poor is most pervasive and pernicious.' It is this divide that, fourteen

years after Mann left Africa, threatens to swallow up 25 million lives in Africa."

Edwin had titled his speech, the "Deafening Silence of AIDS." Joep hung on every word.

The epidemic in South Africa was picking up speed. Thirty-six million people were infected with HIV around the world. Joep thought about the Accelerating Access Initiative, the partnership between drug companies and the United Nations that had just been announced, and hoped it would spring into action soon. But he wasn't convinced that governments would act quickly enough. Some were not acting at all. There was no time to wait, no time to watch them roll out the same, tired models of aid and development.

Everything about this disease was unprecedented: its scale, its speed, the way it shoved a magnifying glass over the cracks in society and amplified the injustices. So why should the response be conventional? This question sparked a new venture for Joep, one that would blossom the moment he returned home to Amsterdam.

But first, there were five more days of conference to attend. More activist demonstrations against drug companies where men and women dressed as the Grim Reaper staged "die-ins," their bodies blocking the ground in front of the company's stands. There were more presentations about the latest science, the newest trends. Joep shoved the conference catalogue—which was as thick as a small city's phone book—into his black backpack and flitted from room to room, dipping in and out of sessions, leaning against the back wall and sneaking out the moment he was bored. He liked speakers who could rouse an audience and stir his emotions.

One of the exciting developments announced at the conference was a new class of drugs that blocked HIV from entering T helper cells. They were known as entry inhibitors or fusion inhibitors and they latched onto one of the leaves flapping on HIV's coat and blocked the virus from attaching to human cells.

The second buzz was about a strange, new treatment strategy that involved taking people off HIV medicines. Dr. Anthony S. Fauci, head of the NIH division that studied AIDS, gave a talk about one of his experiments. He let a small group of patients take short breaks from their HIV pills. Some took their medicines for a month and stopped for a month and then started again, others did one week on and one week off. Tony, as most people called him, wanted to see if they stayed healthy with what he called structured treatment interruptions and if the strategy got rid of any of the resistant strains of virus.

HIV medicines instigate the virus to develop resistance. They egg it on, sort of like a jousting match, taunting and goading the virus—"How tough are you? Show me what you've got!"—until HIV engineers mutations that stop the drugs from working

Fauci said these resistant strains dwindled when his patients took short breaks from their medicines. The original strain of virus returned. That could make it easier to attack HIV when the drugs were restarted, he said. His strategy also seemed to activate T-killer cells, the immune system's assassins. T-killer cells mercilessly destroy their brethren that are infected with harmful bugs, but HIV too often distracts the hit squad from finding the cells it has invaded.

Drug holidays also meant less time on pills, which cut down on side effects and lowered medical bills. The irony was not lost on Joep. Americans were trying to get off the drugs that Africans were desperately trying to get on.

There was chatter around water coolers and near registration booths about a vaccine made by a California biotechnology company, VaxGen, which was boasting that in one of its trials, every single person who got two shots of its vaccine had produced antibodies against HIV. Those antibodies could protect against infection. Now the company had enrolled more than seven thousand people in trials in North America and Thailand for the first ever large-scale tests of an HIV vaccine.

The conference that began with President Thabo Mbeki questioning if HIV actually caused AIDS ended with another South African president's indictment of that question. Former president Nelson Mandela commandeered the stage at the closing ceremony and said, "Let us not equivocate. A tragedy of unprecedented proportions is unfolding in Africa."

It hit Joep over and over, like a bully laying punches into his gut. The sheer scale of this catastrophe was overwhelming. But he looked around the room as twelve thousand people stood and cheered for Nelson Mandela, and he remembered that he wasn't fighting alone.

When he got back home he was tired but raring to work on his new idea. He unpacked his bag and set aside the conference badge, as he always did, so he could take it to his office. A tangled wad of lanyards and chains hung from his office door and reminded him of all the places that HIV had taken him. The virus was about to plunge him into the world of business.

The unique horrors of the epidemic were forcing him to think less like a doctor and more like an economist. Why pander to a government's sense of humanity when money seemed to be the most powerful driver of action? he thought. Why pander to governments at all?

He was determined to get drugs to the poorest people in Africa, so he started a foundation, PharmAccess, and looked for his first partner. It was Heineken. The Dutch beer company was the third-largest beer maker in the world and employed thirty thousand people across eighteen breweries in seven African countries. That workforce kept production costs low and profits high.

Heineken executives had reason to listen to the impatient doctor, who preferred a glass of Malbec to a cold bottle of beer. He told them to consider their future in Africa. You will end up with no staff and no one to drink your beer, he said. Hans van Mameren, director of one of the company's operations in the region, was listening. He crunched the numbers for himself. "If we don't do anything and say, 'Okay, let nature take its toll,' then within seven years, twenty percent of your senior management is gone," he told reporters.

The company was familiar with death. One of Heineken's largest African subsidiaries was the Bralirwa brewery in Rwanda. It sat among banana palms on the sandy shores of Lake Kivu, where dead bodies had floated past during the 1994 genocide.

The men and women working at Bralirwa understood what it meant to lose half their staff in a war. They knew that rebuilding a company and a community after war takes years and millions of dollars. HIV was another kind of war.

Heineken staff in places like Rwanda and Burundi were dying from AIDS by the dozens. In the 1980s, Bralirwa began AIDS education and prevention efforts as staff began losing weight and coughing, their chests too sore, their backs too weak to bend over and stack beer bottles. Brewery managers had been reaching into their own pockets to help employees pay for medical care and funerals. It wasn't enough.

Outside of the brewery, HIV was infecting babies, pregnant women, and young adults. The workforce was being decimated, and Heineken's recruitment pool was dwindling. Joep, as usual, didn't mince his words. If Heineken didn't test and treat its African workers, its billion-dollar profits would take a hit.

The company was already thinking about rolling out an HIV testing and treatment program in African countries, spurred on by the announcement a year earlier that drug companies were partnering with global health agencies to form a public-private partnership to provide HIV care in developing countries. Heineken had the resources, including laboratories, clinics, and money, to treat its workers but lacked the clinical expertise to get a program off the ground.

Joep saw his opportunity.

He had the knowledge and the networks to kick-start a successful medical program. There were no treatment guidelines yet, no advice on which medicines to use initially and which to use when first-line treatments failed, but he had experience in the lab and in running clinical trials, and he knew the right people to help him build a treatment algorithm.

Heineken was his chance to prove to his detractors that an HIV treatment program in Africa could work. "We can do this together," Joep told Heineken executives. "Your people are dying, but we can save them."

Heineken was on board. Joep's experience treating HIV, working with the WHO, and designing trials was reassuring for a beer company about to venture into the world of HIV medicine. It could be a winning situation for both sides.

It helped that the Accelerating Access Initiative, the drug company and UN partnership announced in Durban, was slashing the cost of drugs in places like Rwanda. HIV drug combinations that cost up to twenty thousand dollars per person a year were falling to a few hundred dollars. Prices dropped even further when generic medicines became available. Some combinations cost three hundred dollars a year, a price still out of reach of most Rwandan brewery staff, but the deep discounts helped Joep make a compelling argument to Heineken that it should pick up the bill.

In 2001, PharmAccess and Heineken launched the Heineken Workplace Program. It started in Rwanda and expanded to Heineken breweries and subsidiaries in Burundi, the Democratic Republic of the Congo, the Republic of Congo, Nigeria, Sierra Leone, and Ghana, as well as two countries in Asia, Vietnam and Cambodia.

The problems began as soon as the program launched. The first few employees to seek help were in the throes of advanced AIDS. They died quickly and rumors spread through the brewery that the program was useless. "Those drugs don't work," some said. "Look at those poor people who went to get help. They died." Joep's team worked with Heineken's human resources department to reassure staff that the drugs would work if given early. "Those people were on their deathbeds," they said. "But if we can start treatment early, it's more likely to help you."

Still, some brewery staff were fearful of being seen in the clinic in case their coworkers assumed they had HIV. At the same time, Heineken was automating production processes in its breweries in Rwanda and Burundi, which put some workers out of a job. The timing was terrible. It looked like a purging of HIV-positive workers. "No, no," the brewery managers pleaded. "How would we even know who has the virus? The test results are kept secret!" But workers weren't convinced. Few were willing to take an HIV test.

The director of Heineken's human resources department, François Habiyakare, offered a solution. A dapper man who was well educated and a role model for many employees, François announced he would get tested for HIV—in public. Employees came to watch as he rolled up his shirtsleeve and smiled through the poke of the needle. Within months, a third of Heineken's staff in Rwanda was tested for HIV.

There were different problems in Nigeria. A government-imposed tax on medicine added a 20 percent import duty to the cost of flying HIV medicines into the country. In Sierra Leone, there was no way to test Heineken employees for HIV. They gave blood samples, but their blood had to be flown out of the country to labs in Nigeria, meaning they had to beg airlines to transport potentially infectious samples.

But the program powered on; Joep was not willing to fail. Drs. Vincent Janssens and Tobias Rinke de Wit from PharmAccess managed the day-to-day logistics, and hundreds of Heineken staff, their spouses, and their children came forward for testing and were started on HIV medicines.

The program's first line of treatment cost five hundred dollars a year per person and if that failed, because of resistance or side effects, they switched to a second-line combination that cost fifteen hundred dollars. Annual lab work cost another hundred dollars or so per person.

Joep was improvising. He was picking up the phone and calling Sven Danner back in Amsterdam, weighing the pros and cons of various drug regimens. Which treatments should they use? he asked his old friend, Peter Reiss.

After long conversations about resistance, side effects, and cost, Joep decided to treat with a combination of lamivudine and zidovudine for men and a combination of lamivudine and nevirapine for women. But women who had already taken nevirapine to prevent HIV being passed to their babies were given indinavir instead. This was his plan for first-line treatment. If that failed, Heineken staff and their families were given a different combination using didanosine and other drugs.

Joep's Heineken HIV treatment program pioneered some of the first guidelines for the treatment of HIV in Africa. Doctors from Rwanda and Burundi flew to Nairobi to meet with doctors from the Netherlands, Belgium, and France to learn about Joep's treatment plan—Burundi was considered too unsafe for their meeting. During a three-day workshop, they talked about the life cycle of HIV, the way various medicines attacked the virus, and which side effects to look out for.

Their common language was French, which Joep spoke—with his hands and feet. He gestured wildly as he searched for the right word, cycling through phrases in Dutch and English, struggling to find the right words in French. Joep wanted to speak faster than his command of the language allowed. There was so much material to cover, so many new ideas to share, so much he needed to say. Absent the exact word he was looking for in French, Joep jumped up and down in exasperation to a room of bemused, multilingual doctors.

After the workshop, there was a three-week practical traineeship where doctors from Rwanda and Burundi worked under the supervision of HIV physicians, after which there were twice-monthly teleconferences to talk through problems and progress. PharmAccess asked to start an electronic database to monitor African patients, but Heineken executives were not keen on the idea of collecting medical information. "We are beer producers. We don't need data," Heineken's chief medical officer Dr. Stefaan van der Borght said to Joep. "Let's just give treatment and get them back to work." Joep fought back. "Yes, you do need data! Don't you collect data about the alcohol content of your beer? About the quality of your product? We absolutely need the data to show people that an HIV treatment program in Africa is a success. We need this data to convince the world." The disagreement continued until Joep's argument won over van der Borght. Years later, van der Borght would base his PhD on the data in Joep's databases.

The Heineken initiative was proof that highly active antiretroviral therapy (HAART) worked in Africa. Finally, Joep had evidence to counter the claims made by policy makers who said, "Africans won't stick with the regimens because Africans are bad at keeping time." Look, said Joep, we have a database that shows African patients take their pills just like patients in Europe and America.

When his opponents said African doctors aren't smart enough to prescribe HIV drug combinations, Joep could say, here are Rwandan, Burundian, Nigerian, and Congolese doctors who are proficient at managing patients with HIV. (He added expletives, sometimes aloud, sometimes muttered, always in his head, when countering these racist arguments.)

There will be a quick rise in drug resistance in Africa, some scientists and policy makers said. But by simplifying the regimens, cutting the number of pills, and proving that Africans took their pills, Joep showed that resistance would be no more of an issue in Africa than it was in the

West. PharmAccess started a special study looking at HIV resistance in Africa that proved his point.

When they said that prevention was the only way to deal with the epidemic, Joep rolled his eyes and argued that treatment was a form of prevention. A person on HIV drugs has a lot less virus in their body and is therefore less likely to spread the infection, he said.

The arguments were exhausting, but he had evidence now to back what he had been saying for years. In person, in medical journals, in newspapers, he repeated why it was critical to provide HAART to people in the poorest countries. He had humanitarian reasons and he had economic ones and he was still repeating his now famous mantra: If we can get cold Coca-Cola and beer to every remote corner of Africa, it should not be impossible to do the same with drugs.

Companies came in search of his help. There was Shell, Unilever, and Celltel. Dutch embassies asked PharmAccess to set up testing and treatment programs for their staff in Africa. And just as the world was catching up to Joep's idea, governments began rolling out plans to make HIV medicines available across their countries, and this began to jeopardize his work.

As public pressure and Joep's own efforts shifted the onus onto governments, corporations could bow out and say they would leave the care of their staff up to the ministries of health.

While the Heineken Workplace Program was expanding its reach, the Botswana government was setting up plans for what would become the earliest and most successful national HIV plan in sub-Saharan Africa. Under President Festus Mogae, every Motswana received free HIV treatment.

The year after PharmAccess began to work with Heineken, Bill Gates helped to form the Global Fund to Fight AIDS, Tuberculosis, and Malaria, an organization that would finance the treatment of HIV in the developing world. The next year, US president George W. Bush launched PEPFAR, the President's Emergency Plan for AIDS Relief. It would guarantee fifteen billion dollars over five years for HIV/AIDS treatment, prevention, and research. Also in 2003, the WHO launched its 3 by 5 initiative, which aimed to treat three million people with HIV medicines by 2005.

Publicly funded access programs were being used as an excuse for big businesses to stay out of HIV. Corporations began to ask: "Why should we pay for HIV treatments if governments are going to pick up the tab?"

Joep had to double down on his human rights and economic arguments. Not every public official has the same attitude as Festus Mogae, he said. The war against HIV needs a big and diverse army. The problem is too big for any one entity to fight alone.

By the time the next International AIDS Conference rolled around in 2002, the AIDS community was feeling deflated. After the highs of Durban, the buzz, the protests, it felt like the promises made there had fallen flat. Despite the lofty visions and public-private partnerships espoused from the grand stages in South Africa, two years later, fewer than 4 percent of HIV-positive people in the developing world had access to the pills found in the medicine cabinets of people living with HIV in London and Amsterdam.

Only thirty thousand people in sub-Saharan Africa were on HIV medicines out of thirty million who needed them. And the virus was still spreading fast. Every fourteen seconds, someone somewhere in the world was becoming infected with HIV.

The fusion inhibitor class of drugs attendees had been excited about in Durban was turning out to have the highest price tags of any HIV medicines, and they had to be injected into the thigh or belly twice a day, causing hard knots to form beneath the skin. Tony Fauci's strategy of taking regular, structured breaks from swallowing pills turned out to be a terrible idea. It made viral loads soar and in some cases made drug resistance worse. As for an HIV vaccine, there wasn't one.

The conference was in Barcelona that year and coincided with a few other epidemics. SARS and bird flu raged in Asia and threatened the travel plans of hundreds of conference attendees. Still, seventeen thousand people were packing their bags and heading to Spain to hear these gloomy updates.

Joep was putting off his packing. It was the night before his flight to Barcelona, and he was in an armchair watching the Wimbledon men's semifinals on television. The whack of tennis balls was interrupted by the sounds of Maria and Martha laughing. Anna and her boyfriend were deep in conversation. Ottla had fallen asleep in his arms, and he didn't want to budge, not even when their countryman, Richard Krajicek, was thrashed by a Belgian and the game ended in disappointment. He wanted to reach for his book, but Ottla looked so peaceful curled into his chest.

He was reading more nonfiction these days. A book by George Soros lay on the coffee table. Joep liked the way Soros laid out his arguments and got straight to the point. "He's an unconventional man who dares to call things by name," he wrote in his diary.

Ottla sighed, and he looked down at her face. She was five years old, growing in spurts that seemed to peak when he was not around, which was often. She took his absences in her stride. The kids expected Papa to be in Bangkok or Dar es Salaam and not sitting at the dinner table each evening. They would watch him pack and unpack his black carry-on suitcase, wash a load of laundry, and fold the same clothes back into the bag.

Joep tried to take at least one child on each of his major international trips; this time it was Max and Anna's turn. Both of his oldest children knew that Papa was a frequent flier who frequently missed flights, and sure enough, they nearly missed their plane to Barcelona. As Heleen drove them to the airport, Joep patted down his jacket pocket, waiting to feel the familiar bulge of his tattered passport and wallet. He kept patting. The bulge wasn't there. Joep's passport and wallet were on a side table at home. Anna was exasperated. Max shrugged. It was stressful to travel with Papa, but at least they would get to see his world instead of imagining his adventures from home.

They boarded the plane, and Joep was glad to turn off his phone. It buzzed and rang all day long, interrupting him as he turned the pages of a book or stopped to watch birds dance outside his window. Flights were respite from the constant drain of calls and messages. The two hundred new emails that jammed his inbox most days had multiplied fourfold in the run up to the conference. "Communication, all this communication," he thought. "But who is really considering what they are saying?" Sometimes he clicked "select all" in his email inbox, highlighted three hundred messages in one swoop and dragged them all to the trash can. It felt splendid.

The plane touched down in Barcelona, and he had to dash to a meeting immediately. He was the incoming president of the IAS after serving two years as president-elect, and the society was partnering with the WHO, United Nations, and a Dutch group called Stop AIDS Now. They were trying to scale up HIV treatment in sub-Saharan Africa.

The meeting went well, but Joep was counting down to dinner that evening, when his sister, Riet, who lived in France, and his brother, Jean, who lived in Barcelona, would join him and the kids. He savored those long, drawn-out meals with lashings of wine and tapas and animated conversation with the people he loved. No matter that he had a presentation to put together for an early morning meeting the next day, these were the moments that made life worth living.

Besides, he often scribbled his speeches in the front row of an auditorium, making his finishing touches right as the moderator invited him up to the stage. He had missed countless lectures this way, clicking through slides and checking spellings in his PowerPoint presentation while the speaker before him wrapped up his or her talk.

But this early morning meeting was important, and he was feeling jittery. It would set the stage for the WHO and World Bank to decide if his work to expand HIV treatment in Africa would get their financial backing. Word on the street was that a lot of money was up for play—a billion dollars.

It didn't seem to go well. He was surprised to see so many people in the room, and he had plodded through his presentation without flourish. But at the end of the session a woman from the World Bank introduced herself and said she was impressed.

The conference officially began the next day, but for Joep that Sunday morning began with a tense meeting of the IAS governing council. It was election day, and they were voting for the next president. He had a tricky decision to make. Should he be loyal or do what was best for the organization?

His friend, Pedro Cahn, an Argentinian doctor who worked in Canada, was up against Helene Gayle, the pediatrician who had been invited to President Thabo Mbeki's meeting in Pretoria two months before the Durban conference. Helene had worked at the CDC and was now head of the AIDS and tuberculosis program at the Bill & Melinda Gates Foundation. Joep wanted to vote for his friend but recognized that Helene was a powerful force and a brilliant woman. She was the best leader for the society, he decided. "With a heavy heart, I voted for Helene," he wrote in a diary. Helene won the election fifteen votes to nine. Pedro was upset. "I'm just the little guy from the South, I had no chance against the American powerhouse," he said, ignoring the fact that Helene was often the lone African American woman at a table full of white men. "Pedro turned bitter," Joep wrote. "We'll have to work hard to keep him on board."

The opening ceremony of the conference was supposed to begin with a speech from the secretary of the US Department of Health and Human Services, Tommy Thompson. "Words, words, words," Joep wrote in his diary. Every day that they sat in the Barcelona convention listening to presentations and making the same arguments over and over, eight thousand people died of AIDS. By the end of the conference, fifty thousand would be dead. What good were these predictable, hollow words?

Barely anyone could hear Tommy's words. As he stood behind the microphone and began to speak, a few dozen protesters stormed the stage. "Shame! Shame!" they shouted, waving placards that accused the United States of murdering people with HIV and AIDS.

Joep had been sitting next to Tommy in the moments before his speech and watched with intrigue, wondering how this was going to play out. He wondered if marine biologists or brain surgeons dealt with accusations of murder when they stood up to give a lecture.

Tommy tried to carry on with his talk, but his voice was drowned out by the chants. He left the stage as the protesters were dispersed by security and walked back out to the podium fifteen minutes later. When he returned, so did the protestors. This time Tommy didn't leave. He gave a speech that was probably only audible to people in the front row. Those who caught his words heard him say that his government had increased AIDS spending from fourteen billion dollars to more than sixteen billion.

"That includes a doubling in international HIV and AIDS funding over the same period. Let me repeat that: we have doubled international funding in just 18 months." Tommy could repeat his words all he liked. No one could hear him.

Over the next few days, Joep dashed from meetings with heads of state to cozy dinners with his family. Sometimes he skipped the meetings altogether, preferring to eat tapas with Max and Anna while they talked about their own Spanish adventures.

There was one event he couldn't miss: a reception hosted by the drug company Pfizer. It was a champagne and canape–type affair at the Gaudi House Museum, former home of Catalan architect Antoni Gaudi. Joep walked into the pink stucco building, descended green marble stairs, and marveled at how the IAS presidency opened doors. He mingled with CEOs and bureaucrats, telling them about his work to increase access to HIV drugs in the developing world, hoping he would persuade them to write checks. "And to think I almost said no," he wrote in his diary.

The next day there was a critical meeting with Thai officials about the Bangkok AIDS conference in 2004—the conference Joep would cochair as IAS president. There was a problem. His Thai counterparts who would help organize the conference refused to sign a memorandum of agreement between their two parties. Joep was aggravated that his colleague and current IAS president, Dr. Stefano Vella, was trying to take the lead with sorting the issue. "The AIDS conferences are currently the most important IAS activity; I do not want to depend on an intermediary," Joep wrote. He added a Dutch maxim: *bovendien over zijn graf heen probeert te regeren*, or, "he is trying to rule over his grave."

But when Joep and Stefano joined their Thai peers at a meeting, Dr. Wallop Thaineua, Thailand's deputy health minister, had sharp words for both of them. "If you start a partnership in Thailand, you don't start with text written by lawyers. You start as friends, sitting together to shape the initiative," he said, referring to the memorandum. Joep recalled from his friendship with Dr. Praphan Phanuphak and interactions with staff at HIV-NAT, that his Thai colleagues were rarely confrontational. They must have really offended them, he thought, looking around the table. Wallop's colleagues asked Joep, Stefano, and their European counterparts to introduce themselves "because you all look alike to us," they said. Then they reminded the men that Thailand had always been independent and never a colony.

"We treated them like toddlers and now they are paying us back," Joep wrote. "I am very ashamed of the IAS but at the same time enjoy a Machiavellian pleasure because it solves the Vella-problem. It's clear now he has to go. I will continue to keep him involved but not as the person who is first in control."

Joep told the kids and his siblings about the drama of the meeting that night. Ottla phoned while they were at dinner. "When are you coming home, daddy?" she said. Heleen was driving Ottla, Maria, Martha, and the dogs to their holiday home in Occitane in the south of France, where they owned land close to the Mediterranean Sea. "I have to stay strong," Joep wrote. He was pining to be on holiday with the whole of his family.

He officially transitioned from president-elect to president of the IAS at the conference's closing ceremony. Riet, Max, and Anna watched as Joep spoke from the podium, his face projected onto the screen that backed the stage. "Of all the ills that kill the poor, none is as lethal as bad government. Bad government and lack of leadership has actually killed more people with HIV than anything else." The audience cheered. Anna and Max stared at Papa on the grand stage.

Outsmarting HIV needed precise planning, Joep said to the audience. "We need to go about it like a military operation." And to remind all seventeen thousand of them that it could be done, he used his best line: "If we can get cold Coca-Cola and beer to every remote corner of Africa, it should not be impossible to do the same with drugs."

Bill Clinton and Nelson Mandela were listening. The former president of the United States knew Joep well. He had recruited him to help the Clinton Health Access Initiative expand its programs in South Africa and

Tanzania. When Joep finished his talk, Nelson Mandela and Bill Clinton walked up to the same lectern as he to deliver their rallying cries.

Later that night, alone in his hotel room, Joep wept. He was overcome by the enormity of what had happened and what lay ahead. He had shaken hands with Nelson Mandela. The president of the United States had squeezed his shoulder and said congratulations. Yet there was barely any talk of a cure, there weren't enough new treatments, and he felt a vaccine was further out of reach than ever.

He didn't know, as he fell asleep that night, that in the next few years there would be even bigger disappointments, greater turmoil, and a deepening of the divide between scientists and activists. Joep would preside over the International AIDS Society during two of the most tumultuous years in the history of HIV research.

8 *A Is for Activist*

The fragrance of roasted peppercorns floated from the market stalls. Women heaped spices into neat mounds, red, orange, and yellow powders stacked on top of white cloth sacks next to piles of ripe mangoes. The scents wafted into the air and mingled with the acrid stench of diesel fumes as men on motorbikes revved their engines alongside Mbopi market in Douala, Cameroon's largest city.

Two young women loitered near the spice stalls, their eyes scanning the commotion, not for spices or Suya, the juicy hunks of beef roasted on a stick and served as street food, but for women. They had been given cash and strict instructions. American researchers were in town, and they wanted four hundred women for an experiment.

They had to be aged eighteen to thirty-five years, have at least four male lovers each month, and have sex three times a week. The researchers wanted to study a new way to protect women from HIV, and Cameroon, where dozens were becoming infected each day, was the perfect place for their prevention study.

Forty-three years after a Norwegian teenager sailed from Oslo to Douala and picked up a nameless virus, HIV had spread across the nation. Arne Vidar Røed may have been the first person ever reported to have AIDS, but by 2004, one in ten pregnant women in Cameroon was HIV-positive.

The recruiters worked quickly that day in July 2004. They had chatted to many of the women before and understood how they earned their cash, supplementing mango sales with sex—whatever it took to feed their children and pay for the funerals of their brothers and sisters. They led the women into quieter corners of the market and in hushed tones explained that the experiment was a simple one. Some women in the study would be given a medicine that treats HIV to see if it stops women becoming infected.

Some women would get a pill that looked the same but contained no medicine, just sugar. But rumors were spreading. Many believed the virus killing their friends and families had been snuck into the country by Westerners and spread through a vaccination campaign. "What kind of pill? Does it have HIV in it?"

The pale blue pill wasn't new, it was tenofovir, a drug that blocks HIV's reverse transcriptase enzyme. It was approved by the FDA for the treatment of HIV in 2001, and by 2004 it sat in the medicine cabinets of HIV-positive people in places like London and Miami alongside the dozen HIV drugs available to them.

Tenofovir wasn't on shelves in Cameroon. Too expensive, the government said. Too complicated to get it to Cameroon, some health organizations argued.

The idea of using a pill to prevent HIV wasn't new, either. In 1995, studies in monkeys sent a ripple of excitement through the HIV world. Back then, tenofovir was an experimental drug called PMPA, and a small California biotech called Gilead Sciences had bought the chemical from a Czech chemist. Gilead scientists made a batch and sent some PMPA to Dr. Che-Chung Tsai, a veterinarian in Seattle.

Che-Chung worked at the Regional Primate Research Center at the University of Washington, where he tested PMPA on cells infected with HIV. The drug was more potent than AZT but less toxic, and although both drugs worked to cripple reverse transcriptase, AZT needed activation inside human cells, whereas PMPA was already active.

It was the best HIV drug Che-Chung had ever seen. It could be given by mouth just once a day, it lingered in the body for up to fifty hours, and it took HIV a while to develop resistance to it. Che-Chung wondered if it could block infection as well as treat it.

Brown monkeys rattled the bars of their cages inside the Regional Primate Research Center. They were long-tailed macaques, which preferred to hang out in groups like they did in their native Southeast Asia, where worshippers in temples fed them sweet potatoes and papaya leaves.

Che-Chung gave the monkeys a different concoction. He injected fifteen of them with PMPA, waited two days and injected them with SIV, the monkey version of HIV. The rest of the monkeys were injected with the virus first and given PMPA a few hours later.

Che-Chung tested the monkeys eight months later. Every monkey he had injected with PMPA tested negative for SIV even though he had injected all of them with large amounts of the virus. PMPA had blocked SIV from replicating and stopped the infection in its tracks.

News of the discovery spread from medical journals to the *New York Times*, where some scientists celebrated the discovery and others cautioned restraint. "The proof of the pudding is in the clinical trials," said Dr. Anthony Fauci, director of the NIH's National Institute of Allergy and Infectious Diseases. Che-Chung himself said "it was too good to believe." But the glee was contagious. Imagine if a pill could prevent HIV. It could mean the end of the epidemic.

Doctors don't always wait for absolute proof. Not when they're desperate to help their patients and there's a hint of evidence that something might work. With HIV infecting up to thirty thousand Americans each year, some doctors in cities like New York decided they couldn't wait for a clinical trial to tell them what they felt they already knew. As soon as tenofovir was approved to treat HIV, some began prescribing it to their HIV-negative patients in the hopes of keeping them that way. They were using the drug "off label."

"Here, I know you don't always use condoms, try this. It might keep you safe." They felt bound to give their patients something—anything—to protect them from the virus. Maybe it would work, maybe it wouldn't, but it was better than nothing.

If a doctor wasn't willing to hand over tenofovir, it could be swiped from a friend with HIV or snapped up in a nightclub. Beneath the pulsing bass of house music and the electric blue lights of Los Angeles's hottest dance clubs, party packets sold for a hundred bucks. Inside the silver wrappers were three little pills: ecstasy, Viagra, and tenofovir.

Tenofovir was like a time capsule that took you back to the 1970s. "Taking a T" with a shot of vodka offered the freedom to have bareback sex without concern about the contagious consequences. Others used the pills with condoms just in case the condom split. Downing a T meant nights of peaceful sleep, not waking in a cold sweat worrying about HIV.

The idea of "taking a T" came from Che-Chung's monkey studies and from Joep's research at the World Health Organization. When he had given HIV-positive mothers anti-HIV medicines during childbirth, fed their babies AZT syrup for the first weeks of their lives, and medicated the infants as they breastfed, he had shown you could massively lower a baby's chance of becoming infected.

This strategy of treating people before they are exposed to the virus came to be known as PrEP, short for preexposure prophylaxis.

Doctors had been using a similar strategy to protect themselves, not before they were exposed to HIV, but straight after. Poked with a bloody needle on a harried night shift, a panicked doctor would run to the emergency room, grab a pack of AZT, or whatever pill combination was used at the time, and swallow the medicines every day for a month hoping the drugs would block any HIV inside the wound from causing permanent infection.

If taken within a few hours after exposure to the virus, the medicines lowered the chance of becoming infected by 80 percent. This idea was known as PEP, short for postexposure prophylaxis, and it came into play soon after AZT was approved in 1987, even though it was years before there was proof it worked.

Joep wrote about PEP and how it didn't always work. In an article in the *New England Journal of Medicine* in 1990, he, along with Peter Reiss, Jaap Goudsmit, and others, wrote about "the aftermath of a tragic accident" in their hospital. A fifty-eight-year-old man was recovering from surgery when he was given an injection using a needle that contained a drop of blood from another patient. That patient was very sick with HIV. The accident was noticed within minutes, and doctors hurried to give the fifty-eight-year-old AZT. Forty-five minutes after he had been injected with HIV, he received his first dose of AZT, followed by doses every few hours for weeks. It didn't work. Joep and his colleagues found HIV in the man's blood thirty days after the accident.

In the early 2000s, there was no evidence that swallowing tenofovir before sex would stop a person becoming infected with HIV. Clinical trials were needed to prove it. Seeing Che-Chung's monkey studies, researchers from San Francisco to Sydney rushed to apply for money to run those trials. Tenofovir wasn't even one month old when two proposals to test the medicine as PrEP landed on the desk of Dr. Helene Gayle, the pediatrician whom Joep had voted for as incoming president of the International AIDS Society.

Helene was director of the Gates Foundation's HIV, TB, and reproductive health program, and she was interested in supporting a PrEP trial because a pill to prevent HIV could be lifesaving for women who weren't able to negotiate safer sex.

The proposals that landed on her desk came from scientists at the University of New South Wales in Australia and a North Carolina nonprofit called Family Health International. FHI wanted to run trials in West Africa and Asia, and Helene asked the two groups to work together on the study in Asia, but the collaboration lasted only a few months before it fell apart.

It was a sign of things to come. The tenofovir PrEP trials would explode into a messy, painful milestone in HIV research and a lesson in how not to plan clinical trials. Joep didn't know at the time that the saga would play out under his watch and jeopardize the future of HIV research. Discoveries of new drugs and ways to prevent HIV were on the line.

Turning down Helene's offer, the Australian team, led by John Kaldor, partnered with Kimberly Page's team at the University of California at San Francisco. They wanted to test tenofovir on nearly a thousand sex workers in Cambodia, but before they could secure millions of dollars in funding and get to work there were a few ethical conundrums to juggle.

Such as, why were poor women, most of them sex workers, being asked to test a drug that wasn't available as treatment in their country? Were these women, many of whom lived on the margins of society, in a position to consent to being the subject of an experiment? What would happen if they became HIV-positive during the trial? What if they stopped using condoms and became pregnant?

Helene called for a meeting in her Seattle office in November 2001 to discuss these concerns. Representatives from FHI, the CDC, and other public health agencies, and an ethicist from Johns Hopkins University convened around a table. Gilead sent two of its senior staff. Its drug was at the center of a growing controversy, but the company wasn't that interested in PrEP. Prevention didn't seem like a big money maker when there were millions of people with HIV who needed treatment. The company was focused on pricing and access issues but said it would support the trials by providing the pills.

It was a heated debate that would be remembered as positively tame compared to what was to come. But they could agree on one thing: it was unethical to test the drug for safety in women from poorer countries. Safety studies should be done in places where medical care is at hand if things go wrong. The CDC agreed to run a tenofovir safety trial in Atlanta among men who have sex with men. FHI, led by Dr. Ward Cates, conceded that this was a good idea but added that, one way or another, testing a drug on people at high risk of HIV would always include working with society's most vulnerable communities. There was no way around that.

By early 2003, both sets of researchers had secured millions of dollars in funding. FHI received six and a half million dollars from the Bill & Melinda Gates Foundation to run trials in high-risk women in Cameroon, Nigeria, and Ghana. The NIH gave Kimberly and John just over two million dollars for a study in Cambodia. With money in hand, both teams were ready to go. And both were about to run into massive trouble.

Meanwhile, Joep had moved the International AIDS Society's headquarters from Stockholm to Geneva and was busy turning the society into a more professional organization. And he had started a new initiative called the Industry Liaison Forum, or ILF. He was frustrated that the only thing being asked of drug companies was money and medicine. They had expertise, and he wanted to reposition their priorities and get them to do state-of-the-art trials in the developing world.

No use testing a drug in Nebraska and then giving it to someone in Nairobi, he said. People's genetics are different, their environments are different, and all of these things impact how a drug works or doesn't work. Besides, some HIV drugs have to be taken three times a day with a meal each time. That wasn't possible in parts of Africa and Asia. How were these drugs supposed to save people there?

Jacqueline was coordinator for the ILF. She could manage Joep's anger when some drug company executives refused to attend the meetings and convince the executives they needed to be in the room. She invited them to pair their scientists with scientists in the developing world, people like Dr. Elly Katabira in Uganda and Dr. Papa Salif Sow in Senegal, researchers who had the clinical expertise and the local know-how to make sure drug trials would be designed properly and that the right research questions would be asked at the outset.

Drug companies were confused at first. Forty executives met with Joep in a Chicago conference room at the launch of the ILF, their backs stiff, arms crossed against their chests. "Wait, so you're not just asking us to increase access?"

No, said Joep. What use is access if we don't understand how the drugs work in Africans? We need to build infrastructure in the developing world and tailor the trials and the medicines to the people who need them most. It was unacceptable to him that drug companies helicoptered in to the developing world to test their drugs on poor people and left the moment they had the data they needed to get their drugs approved.

You should stick around after your studies, Joep said, and promise the people who take part in your experiments at least two years of posttrial health care. And trials should be done in countries that have national HIV treatment programs. Otherwise, people were given high-tech treatments while they were enrolled in trials but left with nothing when scientists checked out of their hotels and flew back to America or Europe with hard drives full of study results. Power needed to be shifted, and he was determined to use his platform as IAS president to do that.

Back in Douala and Phnom Penh, preparations were being made to get the trials started. Recruitment wouldn't begin until the next year, but in September 2003, researchers sat down with local women and in one-on-one interviews they asked questions about their sex lives, income, and personal beliefs. They hoped that by gathering this data the actual trials would run smoothly.

Research shifted to recruitment in Cameroon in the summer of 2004, and it was at this time that a pair of activists arrived in Douala. Fabrice Pilorge and Regis Samba-Kounzi were members of Act Up–Paris, and they were on a three-week trip to Cameroon to monitor HIV studies funded by the French government. They were dedicating the July issue of their newsletter, *Protocol Sud*, to Cameroon's HIV epidemic.

The tenofovir prevention trial wasn't on their list of studies to check, but they heard about the trial through two local activists, Calice and Jean-Marie Talom from the group, Réseau Ethique Droit et Santé, or REDS. One of their group's founders knew a woman who became infected with HIV during a clinical trial in the 1990s. The trial was studying the spermicidal lubricant, nonoxynol-9, to see if it protected against HIV, but the opposite turned out to be true. Nonoxynol-9 irritated and inflamed the lining of the vagina and anus—even causing small ulcers if used regularly—the irritation and ulcers helped HIV enter the body.

Now activists at REDS were worried about Cameroonian women being recruited for the tenofovir PrEP trial. Would they be given HIV medicines if they became infected during the trial? Would they be given female condoms? Joep had done a study in four Thai brothels in 1998 that found that some sex workers and their clients preferred female condoms to male condoms.

The activists put their questions to FHI but weren't impressed with the answers. They didn't know that a similar controversy was unfolding in Cambodia and that the future of HIV research was on the line.

In 1998, Cambodian sex workers were under attack. With rates of HIV soaring, the Cambodian government launched the "100% Condom Use Programme" which mandated the use of condoms by sex workers. It also mandated that sex workers carry ID cards. So while HIV transmission in brothels decreased, abuse of sex workers increased. The ID cards made it easier for policemen to find, threaten, and abuse them. Nine out of ten sex workers said they had been robbed by police, more than half were raped by an officer.

Two years later, scared and tired of the abuse, the sex workers formed a union, the Women's Network for Unity—just in time for a fresh round of assaults. In 2003, when US president George W. Bush launched PEPFAR, promising fifteen billion dollars for HIV treatment over five years, it carried with it a brutal provision. PEPFAR money could only go to organizations that explicitly opposed sex work.

The Prostitution Pledge, as it came to be known, caused deep rifts between sex workers and the NGOs that supported them. At least half a dozen groups in Phnom Penh signed the Prostitution Pledge, took PEPFAR money, and stopped working with WNU. Among the few NGOs that remained, rivalries grew, and sex workers were skeptical about their agenda.

So when researchers from the United States and Australia arrived in Phnom Penh in 2003 to ask sex workers questions about their personal lives in preparation for some experiments, Cambodian women had their own questions. Who said you could do this experiment here? Why didn't you ask us before coming to our community? Are you working for the American government?

Scientists and sex workers gathered at long, drawn-out meetings in Phnom Penh. Many of the women were too scared to speak. Some NGO staff being asked to collaborate on the trial and help recruit women thought their funding might be affected by how they answered the researchers' questions.

There was confusion about the motives of the Western scientists. A third generation of Agent Orange survivors roamed the streets of Phnom Penh—little girls with their hands tied to stop them from clawing at their faces, toddlers with fluid-filled heads too big for their bodies, babies with Down's syndrome.

The women wondered how safe this tenofovir chemical was and why their bodies had been chosen to experiment on. "You had a trial in your country, but you used apes. Here you want to use humans," one woman said. "Do you think we are apes?"

They were worried about the side effects of swallowing the pill once a day for a year. Some studies found people taking tenofovir suffered kidney failure and brittle bones. But there was no way to answer their question about safety because no one had studied the effects of long-term tenofovir use in HIV-negative people.

It didn't help that Gilead had covered up some of the drug's side effects. In August 2003, the FDA posted a notice online saying Gilead had "minimized important risk information" about tenofovir and that the company had "been warned not to engage in such activities."

Even so-called minor side effects like nausea and headache would disrupt the women's work and make it harder to earn a living. WNU asked the researchers to give health insurance to women in the trial for thirty years—not for their general health but to cover any problems caused by tenofovir. The NIH said no. Its money was not to be used for anything except research.

The women were also concerned that sex workers in the trial, some of whom would be taking a placebo, might assume they were protected from HIV. At WNU meetings, some said they would join the trial to earn more money because they could stop using condoms with clients. One sex worker told a journalist at the *Cambodia Daily* newspaper that "sex workers in another country had proven that after taking the drug they 'could become free of AIDS.'" She added, "Condoms could prevent liver and kidney problems."

Most HIV studies enroll people who are already infected. But prevention studies, like this one, recruit healthy people and wait to see if they fall sick. The women wondered: you want to give us a pill to see if it stops us getting HIV because you believe the pill works. Then why are you giving half of us a sugar pill?

Condoms and counseling were an integral part of the trial, but the women were skeptical that anyone was concerned for their safety. "First you try this medicine on one of your own sisters, and then you can come and give it to us."

They weren't satisfied with the responses they got from the trial leaders, so they did something no group of sex workers in Cambodia had ever done. They organized a press conference.

On March 29, 2004, in front of stunned trial researchers and the media, Kao Tha, WNU's president, spoke on behalf of its members. "They said they don't want to try the drug because they are poor and they are sex workers... If they fall ill, who will look after their mothers, children, sisters or brothers? If the researchers are so sure that this drug is safe for HIV-negative women to take, in the short and long term, why won't they commit to insurance for us and our families? If we get sick or can't work it can be the difference between life and death for our families."

In Phnom Penh and Douala, activists and community members were asking the same question: Why should poor, brown women bear the burden of testing pills? Why should rich white people benefit from trials they don't take part in? They felt sure that if tenofovir was ever approved to prevent HIV, Cameroonians and Cambodians would be the last to receive it.

Joep was jotting down notes behind the grand stage in the convention center. The IAS had pushed for the 2004 conference to be in Bangkok, moving it from Toronto, where it was originally planned. Since Durban, they wanted to rotate the conference between a developed country and a developing one, and Joep was glad he got to host the conference in Thailand. For the first time in IAS history, the conference hosted a Global Village, including talks and art exhibitions that were open to the public, as well as a youth program giving voice to children and teens who had ideas about how to fight the epidemic.

Asia offered a chance to reimagine the epidemic. One in every four people newly infected with HIV lived in the region, and the Thai government was fighting back against the virus. Here, there was opportunity to prevent further infections, to slow the outbreak, and protect newborns.

Joep loved Thailand, loved to see Praphan, Praphan's daughter Nittaya, Jintanat, and their colleagues at HIV-NAT. He wanted to showcase their work and the government's bold and successful HIV prevention programs. Thailand had scaled up treatment as prevention and was giving pregnant women medicines to stop babies being born with the infection.

But there was a dark side.

The year before the conference, the Thai government declared war on drug users. Thousands were murdered and arrested, even ambushed as they walked out of HIV trial sites in Bangkok and Chiang Mai. Police hid near clinic entrances, assuming drug users were enrolled in the studies, pounced, and put them in prison.

Joep wanted the Bangkok conference to shine a light on the country's prevention policies while shaming the government into ending its war on drug users. IAS conferences were always organized with local officials, and this conference was no different. But working with the Thai government had been a nightmare.

He was fighting for drug users to speak at the opening ceremony, to share their story with the twenty thousand attendees, to have their voice heard. Half of Thailand's drug users were infected with HIV.

Thai officials wouldn't allow it. There was no way they would share their platform with people who injected drugs. Joep pleaded and pushed. Eventually they said yes but the speaker, an HIV-positive man who was a former injecting drug user, would have to speak last.

Sensing something was awry, the two penultimate speakers of the opening ceremony agreed to cancel their talks so that Paisan Suwannawong wouldn't be relegated to the final spot. But as Paisan stepped up to the podium, it was too late.

He wore a black t-shirt, his black hair tied in a ponytail. Paisan was thirty-eight, director of the Thai Treatment Action Group, and he was HIV-positive. He told the audience he was infected with HIV when he shared a needle in a Bangkok prison. He landed in that prison because police arrested anyone found with needles or drugs. On the streets and inside prison cells, fear of being caught with a syringe meant drug users hoarded a few syringes and shared them.

"I got arrested at least twenty times," Paisan said. "Most of the time, I did not have any drugs on me. The police would plant drugs on me and force me to confess, and beat me if I did not sign their document. I could not carry a needle around, because if the police arrested me, the charge would be more serious."

Nelson Mandela, UN secretary-general Kofi Annan, Miss Universe Jennifer Hawkins, and twenty thousand people listened as Paisan spoke about his life in the slum and the brutality of the government's crusade against drug users.

And then, just as Paisan was getting started, Thai prime minister Thaksin Shinawatra and other government officials stood up en masse and began to walk out of the grand ballroom. Joep was horrified. They were turning their backs on the country's most vulnerable people and on their agreement with him. To make matters worse, the audience—thinking the ceremony must have ended if government officials were leaving—started grabbing their bags and getting out of their chairs.

US government officials tricked him, too. After the drama of the Barcelona conference, where Tommy Thompson, the secretary for the US Department of Health and Human Services, was heckled by activists, the US government told Joep they wouldn't give any money to help support the Bangkok conference. Joep pleaded, and they changed their mind. Then they reversed the decision.

Would they at least send an official to represent the United States? he asked. But they wanted assurances that activists would not chant over their officials. Fine, said Joep, brokering a deal between activist groups who agreed to hold up signs but not shout over speakers.

So when the head of PEPFAR stood to speak and a few dozen activists shouted "Murderer!" and drowned out his voice, Joep rubbed his temples and tried not to scream.

Jacqueline tried to calm him. She was rubbing her ears, they were still ringing from the international phone calls she had fielded day and night in the months leading up to the conference, but no matter how hard she tried to shake the ringing or Joep's fury, she couldn't placate him.

It was a disaster. On his stage, under his presidency, a public spectacle of badly behaved government officials and activists was playing out. And yet, these were minor ordeals in comparison to the drama about to unfold.

Feeling blindsided and ignored about the tenofovir PrEP trials in Cambodia and Cameroon, WNU had reached out to Act Up–Paris and REDS. They had heard about each other's struggles and agreed to meet at the Bangkok conference, where they huddled and hatched a plan—they would zap.

A zap was a trademark Act Up–Paris protest, a flash mob of AIDS activists that would descend on a drug company's booth in the exhibition hall or on the steps of a government agency. The Bangkok zap required white paper, black markers, and copious tubs of red paint.

They zapped on day four of the conference. A few dozen activists marched into the exhibition hall and chanted: "Gilead are murderers! Gilead infects women with HIV!" They flung red paint at the Gilead logo, poured it over the stand, and plastered white cards printed with "Tenofovir Makes Me Sick" and "Gilead Wants Us HIV+" onto the walls. Fake blood dripped down onto the floor. Gilead staff stood in silence. Conference goers clutched their satchels and stared. They were used to protests at the conference—visible, vocal activism was an integral part of any AIDS meeting—but this was on a whole new level. Bloodier than the usual "die ins," louder than the average chants.

Dr. Joel Gallant, an infectious disease doctor studying tenofovir at Johns Hopkins University, stood to give a talk at the conference and was surrounded by three dozen Cambodian activists within minutes. "Gilead uses sex workers for free!" they chanted, refusing to let him give his lecture.

In sessions where Gilead scientists were presenting the latest data on their drugs, they were heckled, booed, and accused of unethical experiments on vulnerable people. Joep was furious about this hyperfocused attack. He had been banging on the doors of numerous drug companies, telling them to donate their drugs for studies in case they could be used as PrEP. No one had stuck their neck out, he said—no one except Gilead.

"At least they're providing the drug for the trials!" he said. "Why was Gilead heckled? The study wasn't a Gilead study, it was actually funded by the Gates Foundation but nobody heckled the Gates Foundation so it was completely irrational," he said. "There's so much irrational stuff. You have your token enemy and you go after those," he said.

Many activists admired Joep for the fearless way he poked at the status quo and refused to bend to peer pressure, even when that pressure came from the highest levels of government. They respected how he saw HIV as a human rights issue and was vocal in calling for universal access, long before everyone jumped on the bandwagon. But many activist groups refused to accept that drug makers were acting in the interests of people living with HIV.

Gilead wasn't the only drug company they zapped. Roche Laboratories came under fire for the cost of its fusion inhibitor, the drug that had been talked about at the Durban conference in 2000. Their injected drug cost fifty-three dollars a day, out of reach for people in both the developed and developing world, Act Up–Paris members said. They sprayed "Greed Kills" over Roche's booth in the convention center, striking lines through the "s" to make dollar signs. Roche wasn't doing enough to cut the price of drugs through the Accelerating Access Initiative like it had promised, they argued.

And they were angered at Joep and the IAS for the conference registration fee, which was as high as a thousand dollars in a country where the gross domestic product was less than three thousand dollars per person.

As the fighting continued on the main stage and red paint trickled over the Gilead logo in the exhibition hall, Joep sat in a corner of the convention center and stabbed the keys on his laptop. He was growing hotter and more outraged. His new medicines rattled in his jacket pocket. He had been diagnosed with high blood pressure, and threats of shutting down the tenofovir trials were not helping.

He crunched the numbers in his head. It was midway through 2004, ten people were becoming infected with HIV every minute, and they were on track to see more people become infected with HIV that year than in any other year since the epidemic began. A new prevention method was desperately needed. How could he get everyone to work together?

He was worried that the future of HIV research was about to be derailed. The PrEP trials were only the beginning. Activists in Europe were working to block a new class of HIV drug from being tested in people. If the two sides couldn't come together, their fighting could jeopardize the hunt for a cure.

Joep wondered if UNAIDS could act as a neutral broker between the two sides, but it was day four of the conference and he was being pulled in ten different directions. Still, he would have to work quickly to bring the feuding groups together.

WNU and Act Up–Paris were also plotting. After their zap became the talk of the conference, they were determined to see the trials shut down—a goal that bothered some activist groups who preferred the trials continue with adjustments.

On the last day of the conference, people filed into the ballroom for the closing ceremony and found a sheet of paper laid out on every chair. It was a joint press release typed by Act Up–Paris and WNU airing their grievances about Gilead and the tenofovir trial. Attendees scanned the paper as Paisan walked onto the stage. This time he was scheduled early in the proceedings. His long hair hung straight and loose, his words were clear: "It is painful to be poor and HIV-positive," he said. "We have learned that discrimination still exists, even within the conference venue. The opening ceremony was designed to ensure that the leaders and the majority of the audience did not hear the only voice of people with AIDS on the program."

Joep's sister, Riet, and her husband as well as Maria and Martha watched the end of the conference closing ceremony from the audience; their hearts ached for Joep. He had worked so hard, slept so little, and the conference was over with so little resolved. They tried to calm him down on the way to the hotel. The next day the family traveled to Angkor in Cambodia's northwest, where they walked among the ruins of a thousand ancient temples.

Back in Amsterdam, Joep wrote a scathing essay in a medical journal accusing the activists of using their HIV status to get away with behavior that wouldn't otherwise be tolerated. "Uninformed demagogy," he called it, adding: "such form of activism is only practiced by a tiny minority, but it has taken us hostage."

A month after the conference, the prime minister of Cambodia was at a groundbreaking ceremony for a children's hospital in Phnom Penh when reporters at the *Cambodia Daily* asked about the tenofovir PrEP trials. "Please don't use Cambodian human beings to test the HIV vaccine," said Hun Sen. "Please test it on the animals...Cambodia is not a trash bin country."

Ten days later, preparations for the trial were stopped. Five months after that, the Cameroon trial was cancelled. Some activists celebrated. They called it a victory. Researchers called it a catastrophe that would kill the most vulnerable people.

By the time IAS brought all the parties to a Seattle hotel for a meeting in May 2005, tensions were so high that two armed guards, both named Jim, stood at the door outside the hotel's conference room. Activists, scientists, funders, and politicians sat around half a dozen round tables in the Hotel Monaco, arranged by country. Act Up–Paris had its own table.

Joep wasn't at the Seattle meeting, but it was representatives from his group, the ILF, who had made the calls and arranged for the key players to talk in Seattle. UNAIDS was conducting its own consultation, but that wouldn't be ready for a few more months. In the meantime, FHI had shut down its Nigeria trial site, and plans to test tenofovir in Malawi were blocked by the government. The only PrEP trial going ahead was FHI's study in Ghana.

It was too late to save the cancelled trials, but they needed to forge a way to test tenofovir in both developing and developed countries. And beyond tenofovir, the future of HIV research hung in the balance. How would they run studies to find a cure if activists defined success as the cancellation of clinical trials?

The damage was deep. In their frustration, Act Up–Paris members had talked to producers at a French news show who made a documentary about the PrEP trial in Cameroon. It was peppered with inaccuracies and fueled conspiracy theories and, although it aired in January that year, snippets of the show kept appearing on the internet, feeding fresh fears that a new trial was about to start in Douala. Distrust of HIV researchers flared.

Joep was nervous about the Seattle meeting because he didn't trust that agreements with activists meant anything. He wished that activists operated like a labor union, sending representatives to meetings who spoke with a unified voice. Instead, disparate groups with different concerns lobbied for various provisions. When members of Act Up–Paris walked into the Seattle meeting room, they demanded that drug companies provide forty years of health care to people who take part in their studies. By the end of the meeting, they were in agreement with Joep's ILF agenda that companies provide two years of posttrial care.

It had taken years to reach a consensus, and in the meantime lives were at stake. "Those who will suffer the most from the misguided ethical imperialism that derailed the PrEP trials do not live in Paris," Joep wrote, "but as usual in Nairobi, Johannesburg, Phnom Penh, and Calcutta."

One HIV news site ran a story with the headline, "Are Millions Becoming HIV-Positive because of Act Up–Paris?" It was easy to blame one group when in reality, researchers, drug makers, and funders each played their part to incite contempt and confusion.

Without the tenacity and grit of activists, "we wouldn't be where we are today, we wouldn't have the drugs if there hadn't been the enormous activism in the gay community in the US for instance, that helped a lot," Joep said. "Just think about what happened, in 1984 ... you can finally culture the virus ... and three years later you have a drug on the market." That's only because of activism, he said.

It would take years for the wounds to heal, but after millions of dollars lost, protests in Bangkok, and the stopping of nearly all the tenofovir prevention studies, PrEP bloomed into one of the biggest areas of HIV research. Trials in Thailand, Botswana, and beyond showed that Truvada, a pill combining tenofovir and another drug, emtricitabine, worked. In 2012, after a record eighteen hour–long deliberation, the FDA approved Truvada as PrEP. Finally, there was a pill that could prevent HIV.

9 *Money and Faith*

Joep's hair was shorter and whiter, the lines on his forehead deeper. He swallowed his blood pressure pills religiously. No matter how frequent his flights, how frenetic his days, the pills stayed in his pocket and passed his lips on time, always on time.

In the early evenings, he wandered from his new home—two floors of a four-story house on the swanky Beethovenstraat, which he bought in 2007 and shared with the children now that he and Heleen had separated—to Albert Heijn, picking up spaghetti and a block of cheese for Ottla's dinner. She was vegetarian, and although cheesy pasta was the best he could whip up, he felt a satisfaction in filling the steel pot with water, setting it on the stove, and shouting into the Blackberry perched on the counter for the fifth and final conference call of the day. The world's leading HIV scientists would have to listen to him over the clang of a metal spoon unsticking clumps of pasta in a pot of boiling water.

After the plates were cleared and half a bottle of wine left over from last night's dinner was drained, he hunched over the dining room table, the gold nib of his fountain pen striking out sentences and dotting exclamation points in the margins of manuscripts. The papers were written by some of the three dozen PhD students he advised and rarely saw. Absence had become part of his allure—the intrepid doctor who inspired a new generation of world-changers while seldom making it to office hours. Students relished time with him whenever, wherever they could get it—

waiting in line for Americanos at the coffee shop on the ground floor of the AMC, around the podium after he had finished giving a lecture, dashing from the hospital to the train station. A two-minute conversation with Joep could spark an entirely new focus in their PhD experiments, shift the course of their careers, inject them with a fresh sense of purpose and drive.

An inch of red wine stewed in a glass near the sprawl of manuscripts. He drank less these days, sprinkled less salt on his spaghetti, and had stopped smoking—barring the occasional cigar after a long, lazy dinner in one of his favorite restaurants.

He told the kids he didn't expect to live past fifty-two, the age at which his father had died of a heart attack. But he had made it to fifty-three, and he was relieved. There was still so much left to do.

He barely talked about work at home, preferring to hear the kids talk about their dramas at school, the songs they listened to with their friends, and what books they were reading. They were quiet now, tucked away in bedrooms on different floors of the house as he sat alone in the kitchen with pen and paper. He sipped wine and scribbled and at one a.m., he scooped the manuscripts into a pile, pushed them to the side, and picked up a novel, letting the words lull him toward sleep.

At six thirty a.m., he was up and out the door, cycling to the Hotel Okura, where he started the day with a swim in a pool with concentric black tile squares. Jacqueline was waiting for him, her head bobbing above the pool's glassy surface. They swam side by side then biked to their favorite cafe, where they drank coffee. Beads of water evaporated from Joep's hair as he sipped espresso and watched the corners of Jacqueline's delicate mouth stretch into a smile. She was telling him about the dance troupe performing at the theater next to her new flat overlooking the Amstel canal, its wide windows framing a typical Amsterdam scene: houseboats gliding through the locks, cyclists careening along the canal's edge, lovers crossing the bridge with their fingers entwined.

Jacqueline's relationship with Joop was over, and her love affair with Joep was out in the open. After coffee, they talked about their visit to the Stedelijk Museum on the way to the PharmAccess office, where Jacqueline was communications director. During that museum visit they had stared at the large abstract paintings of Kazimir Malevich, the avant-garde artist who was one of Joep's favorite painters. Kazimir was born near Kyiv when it was part of the Russian Empire.

Joep was intrigued and enthralled by the pure geometric form of Kazimir's work and how the artist split from the conventions of his day and pioneered a new style of art, Suprematism. While his peers painted icons, Kazimir painted peasants, crafting their bodies from cones and rectangles, deconstructing life to its most basic shapes. He said he was freeing art from "the dead weight of the world," taking "refuge in the form of the square." There was liberation in the way he transformed the complex into the simple, which is probably why Joseph Stalin banned his style of art.

Joep felt an urge to go back to basics. He was thinking beyond HIV to the deeply rooted problems in health care. All those years ago, his professors had told him to stay away from infectious diseases, warned him that the field was dead and would make for a dull career. And for the past two decades, a virus had consumed not only his career but his life. Joep raged against HIV, conspired against HIV, dreamt about HIV.

HIV had been his teacher, exposing the cracks in health care systems around the world, revealing how safety nets for the poorest people were frayed and full of holes. HIV had taken him to Mulago Hospital along a road lined with coffin sellers. It had shown him hospitals in Thailand and Senegal, where he met Dr. Papa Salif Sow, the chief of infectious diseases at Dakar's Fann Hospital. Papa Salif planted a vegetable garden outside his hospital, he pulled carrots and cucumbers from the earth, and prescribed vegetable stews alongside AZT, to nourish his hungry patients.

Joep thought about the next contagion that would creep into their cells and cities. It would prey on the most vulnerable people, people like Papa Salif's patients and those living in nations still lifting themselves out of the ruin of civil war. It would target those who were trapped in cycles of sickness and poverty and failed by governments indebted to the West.

While his peers were patching up the plugs in leaky health care systems in developing nations, Joep wanted to raze what was broken to the ground. His peers were building HIV clinics in places where people died from diarrhea. AIDS exceptionalism and the often exclusive funding of HIV services meant specialist clinics opened in places that lacked the most basic health care. The Global Fund to Fight AIDS, Tuberculosis, and Malaria spent more than half its money on HIV and 15 percent on TB, even though the death toll from TB was close to that of AIDS.

Joep was done with small fixes. He was imagining a paradigm shift in the way sickness was treated and prevented. His new fight was for health care reform in Africa.

When a maize farmer collapses in a field in Kisumu, Kenya, malaria parasites burrowing into his spleen and brain, he will most likely wind up in a bed in a private hospital, since government facilities might be scarce and poorly equipped. A doctor will take his blood, press her palm into his abdomen, and squeeze a bag of saline into his veins. Eventually, she will give him a bill. The sudden unexpected cost of being sick might clear out his savings and leave his children hungry. At worst, the farmer could lose his crops and his home. At best, he and his family will be trapped in poverty while he is plagued with recurring bouts of malaria.

Out-of-pocket health payments make up at least half of all health spending in sub-Saharan Africa, and that proportion was rising. The farmer in Kisumu is one person out of one hundred and fifty million people around the world who suffer catastrophic financial loss each year because of illness and a lack of health insurance.

The farmer isn't the only one going broke. His doctor is, too. It's likely she won't get paid in full for her services, perhaps recouping only half of what's owed to her. "When you see a patient, you don't ask them if they're able to pay, and even if they are unable to pay you cannot return them because they are sick. We treat them by faith," one Kenyan doctor told Joep's team at PharmAccess.

In Kenya, patients in private hospitals typically pay 40 percent of their medical bills at discharge, emptying their pockets at the cashier's desk in the clinic and confessing they had nothing left to give.

The doctor will have done the same at a bank, perhaps the same bank where she cashes her checks, saying, "Look, you know me. I bring my money here. But I spend everything on new equipment and my cleaner's salaries. Won't you give me a loan?" And the bank will say "No." A one-woman operation, as many private clinics are, is considered too high a risk for a bank loan.

The doctor will have set up her clinic with her own dreams and her own cash until a few years down the road, worn by a stream of sickly villagers, the tiles on the waiting room floor will curl at the corners, the ultrasound machine rubbed over the bellies of half the town's women will freeze, and the scuffed microscope slides in her makeshift lab will snap in half. Without a steady, predictable income, she will struggle to replace that equipment, her clinic falling into disrepair, and fewer patients looking for her help.

Joep was determined to disrupt this vicious cycle and reroute it into a virtuous one, words he used in an essay called "A New Paradigm for Increased Access to Healthcare in Africa." The essay offered solutions to Africa's health care problems and won a prize from the *Financial Times* and the International Finance Corporation. Joep wrote the paper with coworkers at PharmAccess, including Onno Schellekens, whom he had hired to lead the organization.

Onno was an economist who told Joep, "A doctor who reads one serious book of economics can change the world." Joep could be that doctor, Onno thought. He was quick to pick up new ideas, ready to overturn the status quo, and with Jacqueline's help, skilled at bringing people on board to fund his ideas.

Onno introduced Joep to the writings of Douglass North, the Nobel Prize–winning economist whom Onno described as brilliant and underappreciated. He had written a book about the Netherlands and the United Kingdom and how those nations had started to develop in the 1600s, a process that led to robust, but varied, health care systems. Joep finished the book in a day.

They took trips together to visit PharmAccess partners in places like Tanzania and Rwanda. By 2005, the foundation had expanded beyond Heineken's Workplace Program and was working with multinationals like Unilever and Coca-Cola.

But those projects—which were helping get HIV medications to tens of thousands of people in dozens of countries—weren't enough for Joep. He was itching to get to the root of the problem. The people helped by PharmAccess programs weren't just battling HIV, they were battling poverty. They didn't just suffer crops of blisters caused by a weak immune system, they had headaches from malaria, crushed limbs from working backbreaking jobs, and they had children with a propensity for all the bugs that grow inside small bodies.

"It's ridiculous to give HIV medicines but not treat someone's broken leg," Onno said, after one of their trips. They were sitting around a conference table in the PharmAccess office in Amsterdam debriefing about their visit. "You don't understand what doctors in Africa are going through when it comes to the business of health," Onno said. "In rich parts of the world doctors know they'll get paid and they don't bother where the money is coming from." The room of mostly doctors and nurses sat in awkward silence while Onno, the lone economist, dissected their claims that everyone should have equal access. "That's true," he said, "but you work in rich countries and you don't think about where your money is coming from. You don't have to. Doctors in the developing world have to understand where the money is. They are much more entrepreneurs out of necessity and survival."

They came up with a solution: private health insurance. Countries like Nigeria and Ghana already ran national health insurance schemes, but Nigeria's covered less than 3 percent of Nigerians and, in Ghana, at least a third of the people were not covered. Rwanda, the trailblazer in health insurance, ran Mutuelles de santé, which covered more than nine-tenths of the population.

Joep and Onno, with the help of their colleague Max Coppoolse, wanted to provide health insurance to Africa's working poor by setting up public-private partnerships that would subsidize their premiums. If they could link international donors with African health insurance companies and health management organizations, maybe they could bypass the problem of those entities not being able to raise capital because they were seen as too risky. And by getting the working poor to prepay for health care, they could help them avoid devastating out-of-pocket expenses—the kind that would bankrupt a maize farmer in Kisumu—while helping their country inch toward universal coverage. At the same time, health insurance would provide a steady, predictable income to doctors who would invest that money back into health care systems.

But not everyone liked their idea. "You're proposing a two-tiered system where not all the people would get the same level of care," staff at a British aid agency said, since Joep and Onno's plan would mean only those who were working would be able to buy into the system initially. "If it's not for everyone no one should have it," they said.

Onno shook his head. "You have the National Health Service," he said. "Of course that's the best solution but that's not easy when we're starting with basically nobody having health care. We have to start with small pockets of change. We can't be politically correct and say if it's not universal then no one gets it." Joep agreed. He felt it absurd to aim for perfection when the baseline was so low. Let's start with something and then see if we can do it for everyone, he said.

The Dutch government was on board to support their idea. "Times are changing," a staffer from the Ministry of Foreign Affairs said to Onno and Joep. "Let's give this a go." In 2006, the Dutch government gave PharmAccess one hundred million Euros to start the Health Insurance Fund in Kenya, Tanzania, Ghana, and Nigeria. The next year, the Health Insurance Fund partnered with Nigeria's largest health care provider, Hygeia, to form the Sickness Fund. It gave health insurance to one hundred thousand farmers who sold their goods at market.

The problem with convincing poor workers to prepay for health care is that the care they're buying into has to be good, and in many cases it wasn't. Doctors struggled to get loans to maintain their clinics and hire staff; they didn't track their cash flows or know how to keep proper accounting records.

Joep and Onno thought if they could loan doctors money and give them business and management training, they would bring their clinics up to international standards and invest, spend, and track their money better. Besides the short-term boost this would provide, the loan combined with the business training would make them a more attractive prospect to banks in the long run who, after seeing years of loan payment histories and actuarial accounts, would offer them credit. They hired Monique Dolfing-Vogelenzang, a lawyer by training, to design the Medical Credit Fund.

Monique launched the loan-giving initiative in July 2009, and the first recipient of its cash was Catherine Booney, owner of the Finger of God Maternity Home in Teshie, a coastal town near Ghana's capital, Accra. Almost half the clinics in Ghana's National Health Insurance Scheme were private clinics like the one run by Catherine. She opened the clinic because women in her town were dying in pregnancy and childbirth at rates that she described as "appalling." Except for traditional birth attendants and spiritual healers, there was nowhere for them to get help.

Catherine's pink-walled clinic offered scans, blood tests, and counseling, but it was crumbling. Paint peeled off the walls, the "lab man" grouched about the old microscope he was forced to peer through. He asked Catherine to buy a new one, but her bank, the one where she deposited her cash, refused to lend her money. She could only afford salaries for two cleaners, two medical staff, and she didn't have enough left over for a new microscope.

With a loan from the Medical Credit Fund, Catherine fixed up the Finger of God Maternity Home, attracting so much new business that she was able to open an entire hospital using the profits.

The PharmAccess Foundation was on a roll. As well as financing savvy clinic owners, the foundation wanted to keep patients safe and doctors at the cutting edge of their fields. In 2011, it launched SafeCare, which trained people like Catherine and offered incentivized quality-improvement programs to match the standards in her clinic and others like it with international clinical standards.

PharmAccess also started the first private equity fund to invest money into private health care in Africa, generally considered a high-risk investment. Joep and Onno persuaded banks and multinational companies to pour money into health care through the Investment Fund for Health in Africa. Their idea was criticized by leaders in the field. The British aid agency, Oxfam, believed market-led solutions didn't work and that donors should invest in government-run programs in the developing world. But the team at PharmAccess powered on. Once the Investment Fund for Health in Africa got off the ground, its first investment target was Hygeia, the Nigerian group PharmAccess worked with to provide health care to market women and farmers.

Joep and Onno's work was being recognized internationally. In 2010, President Barack Obama shook Onno's hand on a stage in Seoul and gave him the G20 financial challenge award for the Medical Credit Fund.

Despite the accolades and the focus on health care systems, HIV was still on Joep's mind. The hunt for a cure had been muddied and stalled by the race to find new treatments, but while he was working on the Health Insurance Fund, the Medical Credit Fund, the investment fund, and SafeCare, he was encouraging his staff in Bangkok and Amsterdam to look for a cure.

And he was still committed to working with doctors like Elly Katabira and Papa Salif Sow, who were at the cutting edge of HIV in Africa. Papa Salif described to Joep the experience of attending an AIDS conference in the United States, where he was one of the few African scientists among hordes of white men from Europe, Australia, and North America. "It's paradoxical," Papa Salif said. "We Africans have the patients but we can't attend the meetings. We need to bring science to the south where we have the most people suffering."

The meeting he was attending was the Conference on Retroviruses and Opportunistic Infections, or CROI, an elite gathering of the world's top experts held each winter in cold cities like Boston and Chicago and known for its propensity to reject abstracts from even the brightest doctors.

At CROI one year, Papa Salif sat with Joep and Jacqueline in the hotel restaurant and brainstormed ways to counter the elitism of CROI and tap into Africa's vast scientific expertise. Jacqueline's pen swooped across the pad as Papa Salif's finger prodded the air each time he had an idea.

They joined forces with Charles Boucher, the scientist Joep had shared a lab bench with in his PhD days, to start the INTEREST workshop, a yearly gathering of Africa's top scientists and doctors looking to forge collaborations and share best practices. Joep nicknamed their meeting, "the African CROI." The first INTEREST workshop was held in 2006 in Kampala under Elly's leadership and attended by two dozen scientists. Two years later, Papa Salif chaired the workshop and close to fifty scientists traveled across the continent to Dakar.

These ideas brought millions of dollars to PharmAccess and the Amsterdam Institute for Global Health and Development. AIGHD was founded by Joep's former PhD supervisor, Jaap Goudsmit, in 2003 under the name Center for Poverty-related Communicable Diseases. Six years later, when Jaap's center was renamed AIGHD and inaugurated by Princess Mabel van Oranje and Prince Friso van Oranje-Nassau, Joep was the obvious choice for scientific director.

He hired Michiel Heidenrijk, an economist who had worked for almost a decade in corporate finance, as managing director of AIGHD. Joep and Michiel often clashed in private, disagreeing over strategy, but Joep admired the way Michiel maneuvered within the constraints of medical research, creating opportunities where people had created blockades. In public, when professors complained about taking orders from a man who had more experience leading investment bankers than scientists, Joep defended Michiel's credentials and the way he dismantled scientific silos.

Professors wanted their junior staff to report directly to them, but Michiel was shifting the structure to make it less hierarchical. He felt like an outsider, but Joep said problem-solving on the scale they were attempting needed people from different backgrounds. Michiel wasn't trained as a manager, so the organization was chaotic at first, but the AIGHD team soon fell into its own rhythm, complementing and supporting the PharmAccess Foundation's work.

A few years later the team wondered if the answer to some of Africa's health care problems lay inside people's pockets: they turned to cell phones. PharmAccess joined with Safaricom, East Africa's largest communications provider, and CarePay, a Kenyan company transforming cell phones into virtual wallets. The trio launched M-TIBA, *tiba* meaning "care" in Swahili, a way for Kenyans to use their cell phones to save, borrow, and spend cash on health care. Health insurance companies began offering benefits via the platform, and clinics saw a surge in patients. People could finally afford to see a doctor.

As chairman of PharmAccess and scientific director at AIGHD, Joep continued to work into the night, sending angry messages from his kitchen table when he felt exasperated by the speed of progress. It was never quick enough. Emails sent after seven p.m. were the most likely to be scathing and hurtful, staffers at AIGHD learned. They half-joked that everyone in the team had been fired by Joep at some point, although he was never serious, only frustrated, something that Michiel was left to explain to anxious staffers the next morning.

Joep and Michiel's working relationship deepened into friendship. They shared stories about their families, talked about religion and Joep's deep disdain for Mother Theresa. He gave Michiel *The God Delusion* by Richard Dawkins, the British biologist who agreed with the philosopher Robert Pirsig, who said, "When one person suffers from a delusion it is called insanity. When many people suffer from a delusion it is called religion."

So it was interesting to Joep's colleagues everywhere when in 2011 the Vatican came looking for Joep.

The Catholic Church banned sex with condoms, declared homosexuality a sin, and in some instances, said AIDS was a divine form of punishment. A cardinal in Colombia preached that condoms didn't protect from HIV and in New York City, Cardinal John O'Connor said, "Good morality is good medicine" and recommended abstinence over safe sex.

On the morning of December 10, 1989, five thousand members of Act Up–New York and the Women's Health Action Mobilization had gathered outside Saint Patrick's Cathedral in New York City, where Cardinal O'Connor was delivering mass. "We won't be silenced!" they chanted as a few dozen stormed inside, interrupting the sermon and chaining their bodies to pews. Cardinal O'Connor led his congregation in a loud prayer that drowned out the AIDS activists. "We will fight O'Connor's bigotry," one man yelled as he was arrested by the police.

And yet, the Catholic Church was the biggest provider of health care on the planet. One quarter of the world's AIDS patients were ministered to and cared for in a clinic linked to the Catholic Church.

Two decades after that protest, the Church had a new pope and a new strategy. Senior clergy had figured out a way of dealing with the AIDS problem while avoiding the condom controversy. The Vatican was using information from a landmark study by a researcher at the University of North Carolina at Chapel Hill. Starting in 2005, Dr. Myron "Mike" Cohen, enrolled two thousand mostly heterosexual couples in which one person was HIV-positive and the other HIV-negative. Mike started some of the partners with HIV on treatment when their T cell count was high and others when their immune system was failing and their T cell count was low. He wanted to see if HIV treatment for HIV-positive people protected their HIV-negative partners.

Mike didn't plan on finishing the study until 2015, but by 2011 the data was convincing enough that he announced the results and proved something Joep had repeated for years: treatment is a form of prevention. Mike announced that early treatment with HIV medicines lowered the chance of HIV-positive partners passing the virus on to their lovers through sex, even if they didn't use condoms.

For the Vatican, this was a way to support AIDS prevention without talking about condoms and without being called bigots. In dioceses around the world, nuns and missionaries jumped on "treatment as prevention." A diocese in the Shinyanga region of Tanzania, an area hit hard by HIV, was partnering with Gilead Sciences to make use of the strategy.

Gilead wanted to test three hundred thousand people for HIV and give medicines to an estimated twenty thousand. It wasn't possible, they figured, to aim for a Western model of medical care, where a single doctor looked after a few hundred patients. The Shinyanga region was rural and hard to reach. The Vatican offered infrastructure and a trusted relationship with rural communities. The Missionary Sisters of Our Lady of Apostles and Doctors with Africa CUAMM were embedded in the region, and Gilead staffers preferred to work with them rather than doctors from outside the area, who would helicopter into the region and leave.

They came up with a hub and club design. A hub was a central regional clinic with an HIV specialist, a lab, and inpatient care. The hub's spokes were mobile clinics that visited the most remote communities. At first, people who tested positive for HIV would be encouraged to get their care at the hub. After a year, they could use a club, where a nurse or a specially trained volunteer would run the usual tests and hand out fresh supplies of medicine.

Gilead's CEO, John Martin, wanted Joep to head the collaboration between his company and the Vatican because he figured Joep was a skeptic at heart, and who better to lead a project with the Vatican? Joep confided in a Gilead executive that this might be his toughest collaboration to date—and he had survived the passionate disputes of the Dutch quartet. "This is going to be hard," he told Gregg Alton, Gilead's executive vice president of corporate and medical affairs. "It's not like you're picking Rwanda or Botswana or some other place where a big project like this has been tried," he said. "We're going somewhere truly underserved."

Gregg and Joep took a trip to the Shinyanga region, staying at the hotel closest to the diocese, which ended up being in Mwanza, a two-hour drive from the area they needed to visit each day. The villages were dusty, with sparse brush sprouting from dry earth. Even at six a.m., it was too hot for Joep to go for a run. Instead, he sat beneath the white canopy in the hotel's garden eating breakfast with Gregg, warning him that the Catholic Church could be painfully slow and bureaucratic.

Gregg was all too familiar. He'd sat through a string of bizarre meetings at the Vatican, where a room full of priests talked about men who have sex with men in the most derogatory terms. They said they supported treatment as prevention but warned Gilead staff that the Vatican's stance on condoms had not changed. At one meeting, a nurse who worked at a medical mission in Papua New Guinea sat through the spiel, stood up and rolled her eyes at the priests. "By the way, just so you know, we all hand out condoms to our congregants."

Joep smiled at the story. "If we can do it here," he said, gesturing to the brush, "then we'll show that it can be done anywhere." He accepted John Martin's invitation.

Joep headed to Tanzania a second time in March 2014, boarding a flight at Amsterdam's Schiphol airport with Tobias, his colleague at Pharm-Access. Impatient, as usual, Joep weaved in and out of the line, pushing passengers and stepping on toes so he could get ahead. He needed to be first on the plane and first off.

The plane was bound for Nairobi where they transferred to a smaller aircraft. It flew west and turned above a gleaming Lake Victoria before landing in Mwanza. A kingfisher swept through the air toward the water as Joep and Tobias shoved their bags into a car. Joep spotted an African fish eagle following the kingfisher and pointed it out to Tobias. The pair marveled at the bird's majestic wingspan, each brown wing longer than their bodies.

On the three-hour drive to Bugisi, a Catholic parish in Shinyanga, their car rattled over dirt roads punctuated by potholes. By the time they arrived at the mission, Joep was tired and thirsty. He was sipping a cool Coca-Cola at the side of the street when he noticed a young boy walking next to a frail old man. The child looked eight or nine years old, his skin was covered with scaly white patches, and his collarbones poked out through his skin. Joep lowered his Coca-Cola and whispered to Tobias, "I have to help that boy. Now."

Joep didn't need expensive diagnostics—the likes of which were not available in rural Tanzania, in any case—to know that Isaac had AIDS. He could tell by looking into the boy's eyes. He scooped Isaac up into his arms and took him to the nearby clinic.

Twenty beds lay under a corrugated tin roof, mosquito nets bunched over the empty cots like cumulus clouds. There were nurses but no doctor, and some of the nurses were sick with malaria and wiping the backs of their burning necks with cloths.

Joep helped Isaac settle into a cot and spoke gently to him and his grandfather. Isaac was fourteen years old, not eight. His parents were dead. There was no money for medicines and no doctor to treat him. When Isaac slipped off his t-shirt, Joep saw deep grooves between his protruding ribs. He left the boy on the cot and asked the nurses for help. He then spoke with Tobias, who had noticed a crowd gathering outside.

News of Joep had spread through the parish. A doctor was in town. Two hours later, a few hundred people had gathered at the clinic. A man brought a sick woman on the back of his motorbike and asked Joep to test her for HIV. They had driven for four hours to see the doctor. There are no test kits left, Joep said.

Tobias watched as the crowd grew. "We're supposed to be writing an HIV testing and treatment proposal," he said. "I know," said Joep. "But I'm a doctor. What else can I do?" Tobias carried his laptop to the small office nearby and typed through the night, creating a plan for Gilead's project. Joep continued to care for patients.

Three days later, on their last day in Tanzania, Joep hugged Isaac goodbye. He promised the boy that he would pay for his medical care for the rest of his life. Then he headed home to Amsterdam to find a cure.

10 Cure

He wanted to wipe HIV off the face of the planet.

Over dinner at a Thai restaurant in Amsterdam, he told Tobias that it could be done. First, he would eradicate HIV in Amsterdam and then in Shinyanga. He would show it could be vanquished in Europe and in Africa. It would mean tracking the virus in each of its hiding places and curing every single person.

There are two ways HIV could be cured. The first requires pushing the virus to low levels within the body and subduing HIV without the help of expensive, toxic medicines that punctuate the day like exclamation points. The second is to wipe the virus out completely so that not a trace of it lingers inside veins and organs. The first strategy is known as a functional cure, the second as a sterilizing cure.

Joep had seeded the search for a cure, dropping clues and discoveries along a path he had worn down over three decades. In the 1990s he revealed that HIV seeks sanctuary deep inside the body, within glands, lymph nodes, immune system cells, and the brain, so that even when a person is bombarded with as many as five potent antiviral medicines, the virus sits safely inside these reservoirs.

As a young scientist he helped expose the way T cells harboring HIV can settle down for a long snooze, threatening to wake and resume new lives as virus-making factories. He tinkered with those cells, poking and prodding, daring them to rouse and release their contagious cargo—a daring ploy he suspected might purge those cells, and the body, of HIV.

His first fight, to develop treatments for HIV and put them in the palms of everyone who was infected, had bloomed into a new battle—now, approaching his sixtieth birthday, the stakes were higher and his goals loftier. He felt he was running out of time.

Joep was working to end the epidemic. Starting with Amsterdam, he planned to rid every part of the world of HIV. Some said he was crazy. "That's ridiculous," they sneered. "Why are you looking for the impossible when you can work on new treatments?" Their contention was no sweat off his back. By now he had become a seasoned fighter. When they called his search for a cure absurd, he smiled. For Joep, absurdity was not a slur, it was a place where genius lay in waiting.

Soon after he returned home from the trip to Tanzania, he launched himself into his latest venture, establishing the H-TEAM, short for HIV Transmission Elimination Amsterdam. The goal was to transform Amsterdam into an AIDS-free city.

Joep talked with his old friends, Peter Reiss and Charles Boucher, the doctors he had worked with in the early days of the epidemic, to scheme a way to rid their city of the virus. If they could make it work in Amsterdam, they would extend their strategy and eliminate HIV across the globe.

The conversations were sometimes frantic, Joep's speech pressured. Other times he was laid back, more mellow than his friends had ever seen.

Their strategy was to diagnose people early, within days or even hours, of HIV entering the body and creeping into cells. Joep believed that early treatment could stop the virus burying itself deep into the body's sanctuary sites, places like the testes and the brain, delicate tissues that had evolved safety barriers to protect against the crazy chemical storm the immune system spewed as it chased invaders.

To stop those reservoirs filling with HIV, the virus would have to be confronted before it made itself at home, and that meant finding people who had been infected with HIV in the past few days, people like Daniel, the feverish young man Peter had met in the emergency room as a young doctor fresh out of medical school in 1981.

Using a slew of the newest HIV tests, scientists in the H-TEAM could diagnose people in the very early stages of HIV infection and start them on treatment the same day, a strategy they called posttreatment control. They learned that starting a person on anti-HIV medicines hours after infection could prime the body to suppress the virus by itself without the burden of daily medicines. And by testing and treating early, they could stop the spread of HIV from one person to another.

In 1998, two years after the advent of highly active antiretroviral therapy, or HAART, Joep had shown that the longer a person stays untreated, the more opportunity HIV has to hide in the body's sanctuary sites. Early treatment with hard-hitting drugs likely stopped those sanctuary sites from harboring HIV like a fugitive.

A decade later, a study in France proved this to be true. A group of twenty people who had started HIV treatment within ten weeks of infection had stopped taking medicines as part of the VISCONTI study. Ten years after infection, the virus lingered in very low levels inside their bodies, suppressed by something other than expensive drugs. Joep's hunch in the 1990s had been prescient. Immediate treatment with antiviral medicines was key to controlling HIV and curing the infection.

After their seven a.m. swim at the Hotel Okura, their skin still carrying the smell of chlorine, Joep and Jacqueline imagined a world without HIV. A virus that found a home among injustice and homophobia, that amplified intolerance and flourished where there was poverty, had to be purged. It would mean a battle in the lab and in the streets, in government offices and in the clinic. And it would take more than his team in Amsterdam.

Supporting young scientists had been a part of their grand plan, an early investment in their legacy. Since they founded the research organization, HIV-NAT, in Thailand in the 1990s, Joep and Jacqueline had helped five Thai scientists graduate with PhDs from the University of Amsterdam. Scientists like Jintanat Ananworanich, the Thai doctor who would become HIV-NAT's deputy director of scientific affairs.

Joep had mentored Jintanat as she sifted through the blood of thousands of Thai men and women to find the handful who were in the throes of acute HIV infection. The detective work was grueling and scientists were telling Jintanat to give up. "You'll never be able to cure anyone," they said.

Joep told her to ignore them. "Don't listen to what they say, Jin," Joep told her. "Finding a cure is possible." Those words rung in her ears as she applied for jobs at the US Armed Forces Research Institute for Medical Science and the US military HIV Research Program. Fueled by Joep's scientific discoveries, egged on by his late-night emails of encouragement, his conviction that a cure was in sight, Jintanat left Thailand and moved to America with her husband and two young children in search of a cure for HIV.

A few weeks before the International AIDS Society Conference, Jintanat was at her home on the outskirts of Washington, DC, preparing slides for her talk, titled, "State of the Art HIV Cure: Where Are We Now and Where Are We Going?" She traced the history of the epidemic, the discoveries made by pioneers who paved her route toward finding a cure. She added slides about Joep's early work, the work of his peers around the world, of the H-TEAM in Amsterdam and what they were learning.

There was the story of Timothy Brown, the man who used to have HIV. He is the man people wait in line for at medical conferences, their cameras gripped in outstretched arms as they snap Instagram selfies. His brown eyes squint as he smiles and peers into the camera. "Timothy Brown and me #berlinpatient," they caption the posts. He is the personification of hope—the promise that science will annihilate HIV.

When Timothy was diagnosed with leukemia in Berlin in 2006, his doctor gave him a bone marrow transplant—with a twist. He found a donor with a mutation on their T cells that blocked HIV from latching on and penetrating the immune system. After two nearly fatal transplants, Timothy's leukemia was cured and his immune system had been redesigned with T cells that refused HIV entry. His body had been effectively flushed of the virus, although Joep and Jintanat wondered if HIV was still lurking inside sanctuary sites.

Jintanat would give her talk on the morning of July 21, 2014, the second day of the conference, at one of the largest plenary sessions, attended by a few thousand people. Joep and Jacqueline said they would watch from the front row.

But first, Joep had to make a quick trip to the United States. His former boss at the Global Programme on AIDS in Geneva, Michael Merson, was now director of the Duke Global Health Institute at Duke University in North Carolina and keen on recruiting Joep to work with him.

They talked about Switzerland, bureaucrats, and Joep's new project in Amsterdam and promised to continue the conversation as Joep left Duke and rushed to the airport only to find his flight to Amsterdam was cancelled because of severe weather. He would have to fly to Atlanta, wait four hours, and board another plane.

In a lounge at Hartsfield-Jackson Atlanta International Airport, he ran into renowned Dutch economist, Jacques van der Gaag, and within a few moments of exchanging pleasantries Joep confessed to Jacques that he was anxious about running out of time. The Netherlands mandates retirement at age sixty-five, and Joep was four months from his sixtieth birthday.

Jacques, who was approaching the age of mandatory retirement, reassured him. "Many people find a way to work beyond retirement," Jacques said. "You still have at least ten to fifteen active years in front of you."

Joep fell silent. There was Isaac in Tanzania, the Vatican project in the Shinyanga province, the H-TEAM in Amsterdam, his children who were planning their own careers, a new home with Jacqueline—the first space they would share—and they still needed to buy art and bookshelves, the novel he wanted to write, the short stories he planned to read, the vacations they dreamed about, the Amsterdam Institute for Global Health and Development, his department of global health at the University of Amsterdam, his graduate students, half a dozen new projects at Pharm-Access. And AIDS had killed thirty-five million people in his lifetime, two million were becoming infected with HIV each year, and he was closer to a cure than he had ever been.

Joep looked at Jacques and said, "That is still not enough time."

Epilogue

The plane is in a tree. There is a loud cracking sound as if the tree is split-ting in two but it is the wing of the plane, snapping like a twig. Hot metal is scorching the boughs and a child is cowering in her basement because a body has fallen through the roof of her home next to a wretched field. And she is alone.

A blue-green bird is twitching beneath the shredded yellow foam of a seat cushion and the drinks cart is spilling its stock. Gin is seeping into the grass, over ceramic plates from business class that have shattered, the black Malaysia Airlines imprint still legible on fragments anchored in the dirt.

A foil-topped chicken dinner sits next to a burning polka dot blouse. There is a label on an unopened suitcase: "If found, please return to Scenic Tours +61 2 4949 4333."

Soft grass is matted in the shape of a dancing man, arms splayed, but the man has disappeared, leaving a bare, yellow imprint, and now black boots are treading over the yellow grass, rubber soles are pacing on top of passports, crunching lanyards, a life jacket, toothbrush bristles.

Warmongers are shouting words: Mistake. People. Wrong. Holiday. Is the pilot crawling? Is that a block of Gouda cheese? Everything is melting. Where is the other plane?

Where is the other ending. Where is the ice clinking in the dry gin and tonic in business class next to a plate of dim sum and a really good book.

Where is the slidedeck with the masterplan for a world without HIV. Where is the cappuccino at the Heide Museum of Modern Art and the missed alarm on Friday morning and the long, long kiss at St. Kilda Pier.

The plane is in a tree. The gold band of Jacqueline's amethyst ring is crushed and hope has fallen out of the sky.

ACKNOWLEDGMENTS

It would not have been possible for me to write this book without the support of Joep's and Jacqueline's family and friends. Thank you Rietje de Krieger, Max Lange, Flip van Tongeren, and Bart van Tongeren. Thank you to Charles Boucher, Peter Reiss, Peggy van Leeuwen, and the dozens of doctors and scientists who offered their time, expertise, and memories.

Thank you to the Mayborn Literary Nonfiction Conference for offering community and a book prize when this manuscript was a work-in-progress. I am deeply grateful to the Mid Atlantic Arts Foundation for awarding me a Creative Fellowship and the Millay Colony for the Arts for the gift of a residency where the first few chapters of this book were written. I wrote the book proposal during an artist residency at Playa in Oregon, and it was at Hedgebrook that my book-writing life began, specifically in the beautiful Meadow House overlooking Mount Rainier. Thank you to everyone who makes space for artists to create.

Thank you to Elizabeth Ziegler, who helped fact-check this book, AWP's amazing writer-to-writer mentorship program, and Jehanne Dubrow, my poetry coach from the heavens. Thank you Bob Mong, Rob Steiner, and R. B. Brenner for continued support of my journalism and writing career.

Deep abiding gratitude to the people who transformed their homes into writing havens, dosed me with masala chai and karela at regular intervals, and believed me when I said I could write seventy thousand words in sixteen weeks: Nina, Ninesh, and Ravishaan, Asiya Api, Hussain Ahmad, Aiesha, and Muhammad. To Rif for telling the truth and for sharing wanky coffee in Hackney. I love you.

Thanks to all the friends who provided support, especially Tristan Brown for cooking brunch, David Alexander for creative friendship, Svati Shah for close to two decades of inspiration and battameez-ness,

Clifford Samuel and Lisa for friendship and perspective. Thank you to Yalini for being my sister. Thanks to Emmanuel for constantly reminding me of the ways women are held back and for looking after Lily and holding down the fort so I could travel overseas at the drop of a hat to report on this book.

To the entire *Dallas Morning News* family, who have been there for me and mine in times of crisis, including after a tornado and during a book deadline. Jeffrey Weiss, I miss you so much and think often about the way you helped edit early drafts of this manuscript with charm, incredible enthusiasm, your weird humor, and so much friendship. May you rest in peace.

Special thanks to Tom Huang—you taught me the micro and macro of storytelling in ways I remember every time I sit down to write, and I am incredibly grateful for that. Thank you for helping me find my voice and for teaching me that not every story has a tidy ending.

To the veteran *DMN* journalists who read early versions of this manuscript and offered criticism and many, many pep talks: Marina Trahan-Martinez (you show by example that women are phenomenal), Dave Lieber, and Dave Tarrant for friendship and precious writing advice. I love you all!

Deep gratitude to Jerry Hawkins for telling me I can do everything and for encouraging me to be an artist. I am grateful for your words and your wisdom.

To AZ and Mobb Deep for helping me power through med school. RIP Prodigy.

To my John S. Knight journalism fellowship community at Stanford—thank you for picking me and for the gift of friendship as I was editing this book.

Thank you, Robin Coleman for being a fantastic editor, and thanks to the team at Johns Hopkins University Press for making this book happen in record time!

Dr. Jessica White, my director of studies at Cambridge University School of Clinical Medicine, and perhaps—unknowingly—my first writing coach, for teaching me how to read a person's eyes, hairline, and fingernails to find their stories.

To mum: without your bravery in 1987 and your contagious lust for literature and libraries, this book—and our freedom—would be a mere dream. One day, I will write that story.

INDEX